Prostate cancer

Balancing the risks in diagnosis and treatment

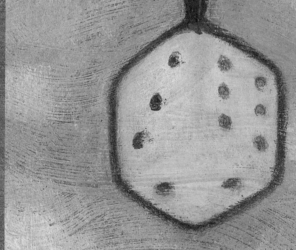

Edited by
Neill A. Iscoe and
Michael A.S. Jewett

THE **CLINICAL BASICS** SERIES

ASSOCIATION MÉDICALE CANADIENNE / CANADIAN MEDICAL ASSOCIATION

Endorsements

The members of the **PROSTATE CANCER ALLIANCE OF CANADA**, an umbrella group formed to implement the recommendations of the 1997 National Prostate Cancer Forum, are pleased to support the objectives of this book: to inform both health care professionals and lay people about the detection, diagnosis and treatment of prostate cancer.

Member organizations
Canadian Association for Nurses in Oncology
Canadian Association of Radiation Oncologists
Canadian Association of Radiologists
Canadian Cancer Society
Canadian Prostate Cancer Network
Canadian Prostate Cancer Research Foundation
Canadian Urology Association
Canadian Uro-Oncology Group
College of Family Physicians of Canada
National Cancer Institute of Canada

The **CANADIAN PROSTATE CANCER RESEARCH FOUNDATION** compliments the *Canadian Medical Association Journal* for this series of articles on prostate cancer, now published in book form. Teaming up with Canadian prostate cancer specialists, the *CMAJ* has created a valuable resource to educate primary care physicians and interested lay people about current and future issues related to this disease.

The **CANADIAN CANCER SOCIETY** applauds the publication of this important resource on prostate cancer. For more information about prostate cancer, health care professionals, as well as patients and their families, may contact the Canadian Cancer Society's toll-free Cancer Information Service (1 888 939-3333).

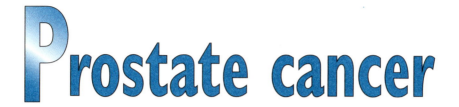

Prostate cancer

BALANCING THE RISKS IN DIAGNOSIS AND TREATMENT

Edited by
Neill A. Iscoe and Michael A.S. Jewett

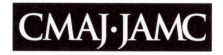

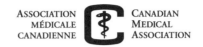

ASSOCIATION MÉDICALE CANADIENNE

CANADIAN MEDICAL ASSOCIATION

© Canadian Medical Association 1999

All rights reserved. No part of this publication may be reproduced, stored in a retrieval system or transmitted in any form or by any means, electronic, mechanical, photocopying, recording or otherwise, without the prior written permission of the CMA or, in the case of photocopying or other reprographic copying, a licence from CANCOPY (Canadian Copyright Licensing Agency), 6 Adelaide St. E, Suite 900, Toronto ON M5C 1H6

Printed and bound in Canada

Canadian Cataloguing in Publication Data

Main entry under title:
  Prostate cancer : balancing the risks in diagnosis and treatment

Articles previously published in the Canadian Medical
  Association journal, clinical basics series.
Includes bibliographical references and index.
ISBN 0-920169-35-X

  1. Prostate--Cancer. I. Jewett, Michael A.S. II. Iscoe, Neill A. III. Canadian Medical Association

RC280.P7P78 1999   616.99'463   C99-900756-4

The opinions expressed are those of the authors and do not necessarily reflect the views of their supporting groups or employers. The information contained in this book is for reference and education only and is not intended to be a substitute for medical or legal advice. The CMA assumes no responsibility for liability arising from any error in or omission from the book or from the use of any information contained in it.

Published by the Canadian Medical Association

Ordering information and additional copies available from
Member Service Centre
Canadian Medical Association
1867 Alta Vista Dr.
Ottawa ON K1G 3Y6
Canada

Telephone: 800 663-7336 or 613 731-8610 x2307
Email:cmamsc@cma.ca

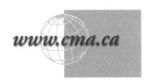

Contents

Foreword vii

Preface viii

Contributors ix

1. **The descriptive epidemiology in Canada** 1
   Isra G. Levy, Neill A. Iscoe, Laurence H. Klotz

2. **Natural history** 9
   Robert K. Nam, Michael A.S. Jewett, Murray D. Krahn

3. **Individual risk factors** 21
   Richard P. Gallagher, Neil E. Fleshner

4. **Screening** 35
   François Meyer, Yves Fradet

5. **Diagnostic tools for early detection** 43
   Pierre I. Karakiewicz, Armen G. Aprikian

6. **Surgical treatment of localized disease** 57
   S. Larry Goldenberg, Ernest W. Ramsey, Michael A.S. Jewett

7. **Radiation therapy for localized disease** 69
   Padraig Warde, Charles Catton, Mary K. Gospodarowicz

8. **Urinary incontinence and erectile dysfunction** 83
   Magdy M. Hassouna, Jeremy P.W. Heaton

9. **Treatment of advanced disease** 101
   Martin E. Gleave, Nick Bruchovsky,
   Malcolm J. Moore, Peter Venner

10. **Palliative care** 117
    Neill A. Iscoe, Eduardo Bruera, Richard C. Choo

11. **Alternative approaches and the future of treatment** 131
    John Trachtenberg, Juanita Crook, Ian F. Tannock

12. **The economic burden** 143
    Steven A. Grover, Hanna Zowall, Louis Coupal,
    Murray D. Krahn

13. **The view from the other side of the examining table** 155
    Ross E. Gray, Al Philbrook

Index 163

Foreword

If you are a man born in North America your lifetime risk of prostate cancer is roughly 1 in 8. Over 70% of men who reach the age of 80 harbour malignant cells in their prostates. Prostate cancer is now the second most frequently diagnosed malignancy in men and, after lung cancer, the most common cause of cancer-related death. If these statistics are grim, they are also difficult to interpret. Is the rising incidence of prostate cancer — which has now exceeded that of breast cancer among women — a "real" trend or an artifact of improved screening procedures? Are we getting better at treating the disease or only at detecting proportionately more "insignificant" tumours? Should we be reassured by the fact that more men live in relatively peaceful co-existence with prostate cancer than are killed by it?

The basic clinical decisions faced by physicians and their patients in dealing with prostate cancer are also fraught with ambiguity. Prostate-specific antigen screening offers early detection, but does this lead to improved survival? In the absence of randomized controlled trials of surgery and radiotherapy, what do we know about the relative effectiveness of these interventions, either of which may exact the heavy price of erectile dysfunction or urinary incontinence? How do physicians help patients balance an improved chance of survival with quality of life as they make choices about screening, treatment and the management of side effects?

We asked Dr. Neill A. Iscoe, medical oncologist with the Toronto–Sunnybrook Regional Cancer Centre, and Dr. Michael A.S. Jewett, chair of the Division of Urology at the University of Toronto, to bring some clarity to these questions. They drew together leading clinicians and researchers to create a series of articles on all aspects of prostate cancer under the banner of the *Canadian Medical Association Journal*'s Clinical Basics series. Collected here in one volume, these articles provide a current and authoritative overview of topics ranging from epidemiology, prevention, diagnosis and management to the future of therapy and patient perspectives. We are confident that this book will be a practical and reliable guide for practising physicians. We also hope that it will be of value to patients and their families, who want a rational, well-balanced and comprehensible digest of the latest in research and clinical wisdom to help them cope with this perplexing disease.

John Hoey, MD
Editor-in-Chief
Canadian Medical Association Journal

Preface

In the words of one Canadian with prostate cancer who has worked hard to galvanize patient support groups in this country, "Prostate cancer is coming out of the closet."

Although it would be interesting to debate whether, or why, this statement is true, we believe that a more pressing task is to shed light on the many clinical aspects of this arguably neglected illness. Prostate cancer, now the most commonly diagnosed cancer among men in Canada and the United States, is second only to lung cancer as the leading cause of cancer-related death in men. If current demographic and epidemiologic trends prevail, prostate cancer will remain a significant health problem for the forseeable future — unless significant gains are made in the efficacy of treatment.

Within the field of oncology there are few diseases as common as prostate cancer for which the basis of current therapy is as controversial. That is not to say that the treatments now in use are ineffective or misguided. The problem is that some of the most important questions in the management of prostate cancer have not been addressed in randomized clinical trials. No practitioner can promote a given therapeutic approach for prostate cancer as confidently as he or she might recommend the use of thrombolytics in patients with acute anterior wall myocardial infarction. This lack of high-level evidence might be viewed as making impossible our objective of informing Canadian physicians about prostate cancer. On the contrary: a lack of certainty only makes it more vital to disseminate up-to-date information and to air current controversies.

In preparing the *Canadian Medical Association Journal*'s Clinical Basics series on prostate cancer, now collected in book form, we gathered together leading Canadian authorities to discuss topics ranging from the epidemiology of the disease in Canada through its detection and treatment to supportive care and palliation. Medical perspectives on prostate cancer are complemented by an overview of the economic burden of the illness and its societal impact. The volume closes with a discussion by Dr. Ross E. Gray, a psychologist who has worked extensively with patient support groups, and Al Philbrook, a prostate cancer patient. They reflect on the earlier chapters from an experiential perspective, which anyone who provides care for men with prostate cancer and their families should always bear in mind.

We would like to acknowledge the valuable contribution of all the authors, who brought to the project their expertise along with a desire to make each discussion accessible to nonspecialists. We also extend our thanks to the staff at the *Canadian Medical Association Journal* for recognizing the importance of this work and guiding it toward publication.

Neill A. Iscoe, MD, MSc
Toronto–Sunnybrook Regional
Cancer Centre

Michael A.S. Jewett, MD
Division of Urology
University of Toronto

Contributors

Armen G. Aprikian, MD
Associate Professor
Departments of Surgery (Urology)
and Oncology
McGill University
Montreal, Que.

Nick Bruchovsky, MD, PhD
Head
Department of Cancer Endocrinology
BC Cancer Agency
Professor
University of British Columbia
Vancouver, BC

Eduardo Bruera, MD
Professor of Oncology
Grey Nuns Community Hospital
and Health Centre
University of Alberta
Edmonton, Alta.

Charles Catton, MD
Staff Radiation Oncologist
Princess Margaret Hospital
Assistant Professor
University of Toronto
Toronto, Ont.

Richard C. Choo, MD
Assistant Professor
Radiation Oncology
Toronto–Sunnybrook Regional Cancer
Centre
Sunnybrook & Women's College
Health Sciences Centre
University of Toronto
Toronto, Ont.

Louis Coupal, MSc
Director, Outcomes Evaluation
Centre for the Analysis
of Cost-Effective Care
Division of Clinical Epidemiology
The Montreal General Hospital
Montreal, Que.

Juanita Crook, MD
Associate Professor
Radiation Oncology
Princess Margaret Hospital
University of Toronto
Toronto, Ont.

Neil E. Fleshner, MD, MPH
Staff Surgeon
Sunnybrook & Women's College
Health Sciences Centre
Urologic Oncologist
Toronto–Sunnybrook Regional Cancer
Centre
Assistant Professor
University of Toronto
Toronto, Ont.

Yves Fradet, MD
Professeur
Département de chirurgie
Faculté de médecine
Université Laval
Québec (Québec)

Richard P. Gallagher, MA
Head
Cancer Control Research Program
BC Cancer Agency
Clinical Professor
Department of Health Care
and Epidemiology
University of British Columbia
Vancouver, BC

Martin E. Gleave, MD
Director, Clinical Research
The Prostate Centre
Vancouver General Hospital
Associate Professor of Surgery
Division of Urology
University of British Columbia
Vancouver, BC

S. Larry Goldenberg, MD
Director
The Prostate Centre
Vancouver General Hospital
Professor of Surgery (Urology)
University of British Columbia
Vancouver, BC

Mary K. Gospodarowicz, MD
Staff Radiation Oncologist
Princess Margaret Hospital
Professor
University of Toronto
Toronto, Ont.

Ross E. Gray, PhD
Co-Director
Psychosocial & Behavioural Research Unit
Toronto–Sunnybrook Regional Cancer Centre
Assistant Professor
Department of Public Health Sciences
University of Toronto
Toronto, Ont.

Steven A. Grover, MD, MPA
Centre for the Analysis
of Cost-Effective Care
Divisions of Clinical Epidemiology (Director) and General Internal Medicine
The Montreal General Hospital
Professor
Departments of Medicine and of Epidemiology and Biostatistics
McGill University
Montreal, Que.

Magdy M. Hassouna, MD, PhD
The Toronto Hospital (Western Division)
Associate Professor
Department of Surgery (Urology)
University of Toronto
Toronto, Ont.

Jeremy P.W. Heaton, MA, MD
Professor
Departments of Urology, Pharmacology and Toxicology
Queen's University
Kingston, Ont.

Neill A. Iscoe, MD, MSc
Associate Professor
Medical Oncology
Toronto–Sunnybrook Regional Cancer Centre
Sunnybrook & Women's College Health Sciences Centre
University of Toronto
Toronto, Ont.

Michael A.S. Jewett, MD
Professor and Chairman
Division of Urology
University of Toronto
Toronto, Ont.

Pierre I. Karakiewicz, MD
Chief Resident
Department of Surgery (Urology)
McGill University
Montreal, Que.

Laurence H. Klotz, MD
Associate Professor of Surgery
Division of Urology
Sunnybrook & Women's College Health Sciences Centre
University of Toronto
Toronto, Ont.

Murray D. Krahn, MD, MSc
Staff Physician
The Toronto Hospital
Assistant Professor
Departments of Medicine, Laboratory Medicine and Pathobiology
Programme in Clinical Epidemiology and Health Services Research
University of Toronto
Toronto, Ont.

Isra G. Levy, MB BCh, MSc
Director
Health Programs
Canadian Medical Association
Adjunct Professor
Department of Epidemiology
and Community Medicine
University of Ottawa
Ottawa, Ont.

François Meyer, MD, DSc
Professeur
Département de médecine sociale
et préventive
Faculté de médecine
Université Laval
Québec (Québec)

Malcolm J. Moore, MD
Departments of Medicine
and Pharmacology
Princess Margaret Hospital
University of Toronto
Toronto, Ont.

Robert K. Nam, MD
Resident in Urology
University of Toronto
Toronto, Ont.

Al Philbrook, BA, BLA
Vice-Chair
Man to Man Prostate Cancer
Support Group
Toronto, Ont.

Ernest W. Ramsey, MD
Professor
Department of Surgery (Urology)
University of Manitoba
Health Sciences Centre
Winnipeg, Man.

Ian F. Tannock, MD, PhD
Daniel E. Bergsagel Professor
of Medical Oncology
Princess Margaret Hospital
University of Toronto
Toronto, Ont.

John Trachtenberg, MD
Director
The Prostate Centre
Princess Margaret Hospital
The Toronto Hospital
Fleck Tanenbaum Chair of Prostatic
Disease
Professor of Surgery
University of Toronto
Toronto, Ont.

Peter Venner, BMSc, MD
Senior Medical Oncologist
Cross Cancer Institute
Professor
Department of Oncology
Faculty of Medicine
University of Alberta
Edmonton, Alta.

Padraig Warde, MB BCh, BAO
Staff Radiation Oncologist
Genitourinary Oncology Site Group
Leader
Princess Margaret Hospital
Associate Professor
University of Toronto
Toronto, Ont.

Hanna Zowall, MA
Director, Economic Evaluations
Centre for the Analysis
of Cost-Effective Care
Division of Clinical Epidemiology
The Montreal General Hospital
Montreal, Que.

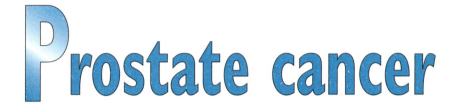

BALANCING THE RISKS IN DIAGNOSIS AND TREATMENT

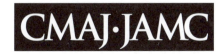

1

The descriptive epidemiology in Canada

Isra G. Levy, MB BCh, MSc; Neill A. Iscoe, MD, MSc; Laurence H. Klotz, MD

> A 70-year-old woman who experienced a long period of depression after her first husband's death from prostate cancer at the age of 63 has become increasingly anxious about her own health and that of her close family. A few years ago she married a man her own age; he is in good physical condition. Last year the family spent much of the winter in Florida, where the woman noticed several stories in the media suggesting that an epidemic of prostate cancer is occurring in North America and that because early detection can save lives, men of retirement age should be checked by their physicians as soon as possible. In addition, 2 close friends were recently diagnosed with prostate cancer. On his latest fishing trip her husband learned from a friend that 1 in 8 men get prostate cancer. He has not seen his family physician for several years, but his wife has booked an appointment for them to discuss their concerns.

Prostate cancer has now surpassed lung cancer as the most frequently diagnosed cancer in Canadian men (except for nonmelanotic skin cancer, which is rarely fatal). Although the number of cases diagnosed annually may have peaked in 1997, it is striking that the estimated incidence for that year exceeded that for breast cancer.[1] Between 1970 and 1990 the incidence of prostate cancer increased steadily by approximately 3% annually. During that period, the number of deaths from the disease also increased, but at a slower rate, about 1% annually.[2] Prostate cancer is, after lung cancer, the most common cause of cancer-related death in men.

Increasing awareness of these trends on the part of health care professionals and the public has resulted in the recognition of prostate cancer

> **KEY POINTS**
> - Prostate cancer is the most commonly diagnosed cancer in Canadian men.
> - A man born in 1993 has a 1-in-8 chance of being diagnosed with prostate cancer and a 1-in-26 chance of dying from the disease during his lifetime.
> - The risk of prostate cancer increases with age.
> - With the aging of the population, primary care physicians can expect to be confronted by this disease more frequently.

as a significant public health problem. An estimated 48 100 Canadian men were diagnosed with prostate cancer during the 1980s.[3] On the basis of incidence trends that predate the significant use of new diagnostic technologies such as prostate-specific antigen (PSA) testing and transrectal ultrasonography, as many as 35 200 new cases of prostate cancer are expected to be diagnosed in Canada in the year 2016.[4]

The PSA test, which facilitates early detection, has been available in Canada since 1986, although its use did not become widespread until the early 1990s.[5] Data for that period suggest that the introduction of PSA testing caused, predictably, an initial increase in the observed incidence as the reservoir of existing, undiagnosed cases became apparent.[1,5]

In 1997 prostate cancer accounted for an estimated 28% (19 800 cases) of newly diagnosed cancer in men.[1] (The number of cases detected annually may decline somewhat in future, once the pool of prevalent cases detectable by PSA testing is exhausted, but it is not possible to predict the timing, duration or magnitude of such a decline with any certainty.) These 19 800 cases in Canada translate into approximately 1 new case per year in every 750 men and are more than double the 9600 cases that occurred a decade earlier, in 1988 (Canadian Cancer Registry, 1988: unpublished data). Also, more than 12% (4100 cases) of cancer-related deaths in men in 1997 are estimated to have been caused by prostate cancer.[1]

In view of these data it is likely that most family physicians whose practice population has an age–sex profile similar to that of the general population will encounter at least one patient with a problem related to prostate cancer each year. Despite the relatively good prognosis reflected in annual case fatality rates of approximately 20% (4100 deaths per 19 800 new cases), many such patients will die of the disease. Physicians need to have a clear understanding of the risk of being diagnosed with and dying from prostate cancer and to be able to communicate that risk in a way that is meaningful to patients and their families.

Trends

A man's risk of being diagnosed with or dying from prostate cancer increases markedly with age. In men under 50 years of age the disease is uncommon, and death from it is rare. Between 1980 and the early 1990s the age-specific incidence in Canada increased among all men over the age of 40 (Fig. 1). However, there was no consistent trend in age-specific mortality (Fig. 2). Over the longer period from 1973 to 1993 the incidence rate increased more than 2-fold, from 60.5 to 138.7 per 100 000 men (Fig. 3). Before 1990 the average annual increase was approximately 3%; between 1990 and 1993 it was about 12%. The mortality rate, on the other hand, increased by only about 20% between 1973 and 1989 (from 25.0 to 29.8 per 100 000 men) at an average annual rate of about 1%. It appears to have reached a plateau during the 1990s; after peaking at 31.3 per 100 000 in 1991, it decreased noticeably to 28.2 per 100 000 in 1996.

The 1993 age-specific incidence rates (Fig. 1) are especially relevant if one considers the future impact of this disease. By multiplying the rate for each age group by the number of men in that age group and summing the results, one can derive the total number of cases that will occur in the population as its present age structure is carried into the future, assuming the ratio remains constant. However, the Canadian population is aging. Fig. 4 shows the age pattern of the male population over 40 years of age in 1996 and the projected pattern[6] to the year 2016.

The incidence and mortality rates for prostate cancer vary from province to province (Fig. 5), but the variation in observed incidence is much greater than the variation in mortality.

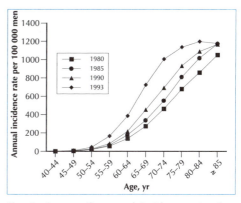

Fig. 1: Age-specific annual incidence rates (per 100 000 men) for prostate cancer in Canada, 1980, 1985, 1990 and 1993.

Lifetime and age-specific risks

The current lifetime risk of a Canadian man being diagnosed with prostate cancer is 12.3%, or about 1 in 8, as compared with 1 in 11 in the mid-1980s and close to 1 in 20 in the early 1970s.[7] The lifetime risk of prostate cancer being

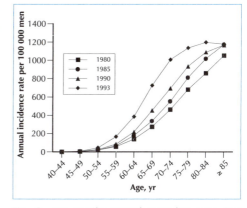

Fig. 2: Age-specific annual mortality rates (per 100 000 men) for prostate cancer in Canada, 1980, 1985, 1990 and 1995.

listed as the cause of death is 3.8%, or about 1 in 26. These data assume that a cohort of men is observed from birth until death at any age from less than 1 year to more than 90 years.

Estimated risks for men of various ages over their remaining life and for shorter intervals are shown in Table 1. Although a man's *annual* risk of being diagnosed with prostate cancer rises with increasing age, his *lifetime* risk declines the longer he survives. For example, a man of 70 has a lower lifetime risk of prostate cancer than a man of 50 because he has 20 fewer years at risk. Also, shorter-term risks decline among men older than about 75 years because the effect of the increase in annual incidence (Fig. 1) begins to be offset by the increasing probability of dying from another cause.

The extraordinary 1-in-8 lifetime risk of prostate cancer in Canada is consistent with risk profiles seen at the end of the 1980s among men in the United States[8] and reflects, in part, the recent upsurge in incidence among men of all ages related to the increased use of PSA testing and related diagnostic activity. It has been argued that such estimates exaggerate the true risks, because with the increased sensitivity of diagnostic procedures many of the cases that are detected are microscopic, "clinically insignificant" cancers known to exist in a high proportion of men over the age of 50.[9]

However, this argument does not speak to the emotional, physical and financial impact of the diagnosis and treatment of prostate cancer for individual men, their loved ones and society. For example, in a recent nonrandom survey of Canadian men with prostate cancer, more than a third of the 965 respondents reported side effects of

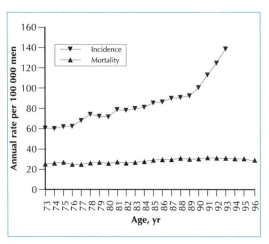

Fig. 3: Age-standardized annual incidence rates, 1973–1993, and mortality rates, 1973–1996, for prostate cancer in Canada. Rates are per 100 000 men and are standardized to the 1991 Canadian population.

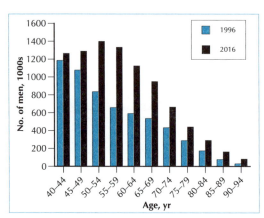

Fig. 4: Age structure of the Canadian male population from 1996 to 2016 (projected[6]).

treatment, and 25% reported incontinence.[10] Half reported that a problem with sexual function had developed since their diagnosis. Erectile failure occurs in 20% to 90% of patients who have surgery for prostate cancer and in 20% to 40% who undergo radiotherapy.[11]

We should also bear in mind that the rise in incidence predates the use of newer diagnostic technologies. As noted earlier, incidence increased by roughly 3% per year in the 2 decades that preceded the adoption of PSA testing in Canada. Although a portion of this increase can be attributed to a trend toward earlier serendipitous detection of the so-called "clinically insignificant" cancers (because of greater use of transurethral prostatectomy for putatively benign hypertrophy),[1,12] there is still a possibility that a rise in unidentified environmental risk factors has contributed to the increase and will continue to do so. The historical increase in mortality rate, although relatively small, further suggests that the higher incidence rates cannot be attributed solely to detection of lesions that are clinically insignificant.

Judging from the simple application of age-specific risks to our aging population, it is clear that the burden of prostate cancer will increase dramatically in the coming decades. The aging of the "baby boom" generation alone will have important long-term consequences for health care delivery and research priorities in the context of this disease.[4] This effect will be independent of, although perhaps compounded by, changes in observed incidence that may result from changes in diagnostic practice.

Predicting annual incidence and mortality rates is problematic. Even today, there is substantial interjurisdictional variation in incidence in Canada (and in other countries such as the United States[13]), probably largely as a result of differing diagnostic practices. The future impact on survival of the current use of early

> **KEY POINTS**
> - Between 1973 and 1993 the incidence of prostate cancer more than doubled. The increase was greatest after the advent of prostate-specific antigen (PSA) testing.
> - Over the same period, the mortality rate increased by 20%.
> - The incidence will decline once PSA testing has exhausted the pool of existing undetected cases, but when this will occur or how significant the decrease will be is uncertain.

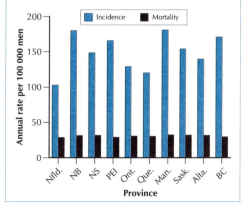

Fig. 5: Annual provincial incidence and mortality rates (per 100 000 men) for prostate cancer in Canada.

KEY POINTS
- A man's annual risk of being diagnosed with prostate cancer increases with age.
- His lifetime risk of prostate cancer decreases with age.

detection tools cannot be estimated.[14] Some decrease in observed annual incidence may occur as the pool of prevalent cases being detected by the first "sweep" of PSA testing through the population diminishes. Such a decrease has recently been observed in the United States.[15] It is also possible that the slow increase in mortality rate that has long been a feature of this disease is finally reversing and that the decrease seen most noticeably in 1996 will be sustained. What *can* be predicted with certainty is that there will be a large increase in the number of men affected by prostate cancer in the future. This will likely be accompanied by increasing demands on scarce health care and supportive care resources.

The Canadian public has little knowledge of prostate cancer and the controversies that surround it.[16] Increasing awareness of the impact of this disease on individuals and society has led to the founding of the Canadian Prostate Cancer Network, a national network of support groups. In 1997 the Canadian Cancer Society spearheaded the first National Prostate Cancer Forum to raise awareness of the public health burden of the disease and to set an agenda for action in the areas of research, interdisciplinary communication and advocacy.[17]

As the prevalence of the disease rises and awareness of its impact increases, primary care physicians will increasingly be faced with questions from patients about their risk of prostate cancer. A table of probabilities can be used to assist in such discussions (Table 1). These probabilities are calculated on the assumption that the age-specific incidence and mortality rates for all Canada in a given period will prevail throughout the lifetime of a man anywhere in the country as he ages. Because these rates may not, in fact, remain stable into the future and because they are subject to some geographic variability, patients should be advised that these probabilities are only approximations to guide discussion.

In the case described at the beginning of the article, the family physician can use the table to assure the patient and his wife that his lifetime risk of prostate cancer is not 1 in 8 but, given his age, closer to 1 in 12 (8.1%). This

Table 1: Probability of prostate cancer occurring in men of various ages

	Time frame; risk of occurrence, %		
Age, yr	Within 5 yr	Within 10 yr	Within lifetime
40	0.01	0.04	12.27
45	0.04	0.21	12.26
50	0.20	0.74	12.23
55	0.72	2.13	12.08
60	2.02	4.41	11.57
65	4.04	7.16	10.25
70	6.16	9.45	8.10
75	7.77	10.45	5.45
80	8.18	9.50	2.88
85	6.71	7.73	1.09
90*	5.01	–	0.38

*There are not enough data to calculate the risk of occurrence within 10 years.

risk, although not insignificant, is also a "long-term" risk. His chance of being diagnosed with prostate cancer in the next 5 years is only about 6%, or 1 in 16.

The table can also be used to show younger men that their risk of prostate cancer in the short term is low. In a group of 1000 men aged 50, only 2 can expect to be diagnosed with prostate cancer in the next 5 years and only 7 will be diagnosed with the disease before they turn 60. However, when those same men reach the age of 75 years, 78 of them can expect to be diagnosed within 5 years and 105 within 10 years. Such considerations may be more relevant and meaningful to individual men of various ages than the 1-in-8 lifetime risk. Family physicians can provide an invaluable service by clarifying for their patients the actual meaning of "all those numbers."

The data should also be of interest to health care planners and policymakers. The burden of prostate cancer is high and will rise. Those most at risk are elderly men, who will need appropriate services and treatments.

References

1. National Cancer Institute of Canada. *Canadian cancer statistics, 1997*. Toronto: The Institute; 1997.
2. Levy IG, Gibbons L, Collins JP, Perkins DG, Mao Y. Prostate cancer trends in Canada: Rising incidence or increased detection? *CMAJ* 1992;149:617-24.
3. National Cancer Institute of Canada. *Canadian cancer statistics, 1995*. Toronto: The Institute; 1995.
4. Morrison HI, MacNeill IB, Miller D, Levy I, Xie L, Mao Y. The impending Canadian prostate cancer epidemic. *Can J Public Health* 1995;86:274-8.
5. Levy IG. Prostate cancer: the epidemiological perspective. *Can J Oncol* 1994;4[Suppl 1]:4-7.
6. *Population projections for Canada, provinces and territories, 1993–2016*. Ottawa: Statistics Canada; 1993.
7. National Cancer Institute of Canada. *Canadian cancer statistics, 1993*. Toronto: The Institute; 1993.
8. Miller BA, Hayes RB, Potosky AL, Brawley O, Kaplan R. Prostate. *SEER Cancer Statistics Review 1973-1990*. Bethesda: National Cancer Institute; 1993, p. 369-79.
9. Bowersox J. Experts debate PSA screening for prostate cancer. *J Natl Cancer Inst* 1992;84:1856-7.
10. Gray RE, Klotz LH, Iscoe NA, Fitch MI, Franssen E, Johnson BJ, et al. Results of a survey of Canadian men with prostate cancer. *Can J Urol* 1997;4:359-65.
11. American Urological Association Guidelines Development Group. *Management of clinically localized prostate cancer*. Baltimore: The Association; 1995.
12. Potosky AL, Kessler L, Gridley G, Brown CC, Horn JW. Rise in prostatic cancer incidence associated with increased use of transurethral resection. *J Natl Cancer Inst* 1990;82:1624-8.
13. Lu-Yao GL, Greenberg ER. Changes in prostate cancer incidence and treatment in USA. *Lancet* 1994;343:251-4.
14. Woolf SH. Screening for prostate cancer with prostate-specific antigen. *N Engl J Med* 1995;333:1401-5.

15. Merrill RM, Potosky AL, Feuer EJ. Changing trends in US prostate cancer incidence rates. *J Natl Cancer Inst* 1996;88:1683-5.
16. Mercer SI, Goel V, Levy IG, Ashbury FD, Iverson DC, Iscoe NA. Prostate cancer screening in the midst of controversy: Canadian men's knowledge, beliefs, utilization and future intentions. *Can J Public Health* 1997;88:327-32.
17. Phillips R, editor. *Call for action on prostate cancer. Report and recommendations from the 1997 National Prostate Cancer Forum.* Toronto: Canadian Cancer Society; 1997.
18. Zdeb MS. The probability of developing cancer. *Am J Epidemiol* 1977;106:6-16.
19. Seidman H, Silverberg E, Bodden A. Probabilities of eventually developing and of dying of cancer. *CA Cancer J Clin* 1978;28:33-46.

We thank Howard Morrison of the Cancer Bureau, Laboratory Centre for Disease Control, Health Canada, for helpful comments on the text, and Laurie Gibbons and Chris Waters, also of the Cancer Bureau, for helping to produce analyses and figures. Data were provided by Statistics Canada. The cooperation of Statistics Canada and of the provincial and territorial cancer registries that supply the data to Statistics Canada is gratefully acknowledged.

Appendix: Statistical methods

Annual age-specific incidence rates for the period 1973–1993 and mortality rates for the period 1973–1996 were calculated for prostate cancer (International Classification of Diseases code 185) for all Canada in 5-year age groups. Data were obtained from the Canadian Cancer Registry (formerly the National Cancer Incidence Reporting System) and the Canadian Mortality Database at Statistics Canada. Population data were obtained from Statistics Canada census publications.

Age-standardized incidence and mortality rates were calculated by the direct method for all Canada and for individual provinces using the 1991 Canadian population as the standard. The probabilities of being diagnosed with or determined to have died from prostate cancer were calculated using standard life-table methods.[18,19] The probabilities are based on a hypothetical cohort of 100 000 Canadian men who are subject, during their lifetimes, to current age-specific incidence and mortality rates (1993) and to all-cause mortality risks (1992–1994).

2

Natural history

Robert K. Nam, MD; Michael A.S. Jewett, MD; Murray D. Krahn, MD, MSc

A 65-year-old man consults his family physician because he is experiencing a frequent and urgent need to urinate. A digital rectal examination reveals a minimally enlarged prostate with no focal nodularity. The level of prostate-specific antigen in the patient's serum is higher than the normal range for his age group. Transrectal ultrasound-guided biopsy shows adenocarcinoma of the prostate, with a Gleason score of 6 out of 10 (intermediate-grade tumour). Further history-taking reveals that the patient had a myocardial infarction within the past year and that he has mild chronic obstructive pulmonary disease caused by 50 years of smoking. The man is married and sexually active. There is no family history of prostate cancer. The patient is referred to a urologist, who discusses the natural history of prostate cancer and the treatment options (surgery, radiotherapy and watchful waiting), after clinical and radiographic assessment reveals that the lesion is localized to the prostate gland. Unsatisfied, the patient returns to his family physician to request another opinion and more information about his prognosis if he elects not to undergo surgery or radiotherapy.

To address the concerns of the patient described in this case the family physician must consider 3 interrelated questions:
- What is the natural history of adenocarcinoma of the prostate?
- How important is the patient's age, the previous myocardial infarction and the mild chronic obstructive pulmonary disease?
- Is watchful waiting a reasonable strategy for this man? What about delaying surgery or radiotherapy until there is evidence of disease progression?

Natural history of adenocarcinoma of the prostate

What we know about the natural history of prostate cancer comes from case series and cohort studies in which patients with localized prostate cancer received neither surgery nor radiotherapy. This treatment strategy has been termed "watchful waiting," "expectant management" and "conservative management." Since 1980, 16 centres have reported case series of conservatively managed, clinically localized prostate cancer;[1-16] only 3 of these have reported prospectively gathered data.[1,6,12] Most of the studies have reported the prognosis of patients diagnosed with prostate cancer in the 1970s and 1980s. In addition, 2 population-based, retrospective cohort studies have been published.[2,17]

Methods for assessing prognosis

The quality of the methods used in the studies cited varies widely. The results of poorly conducted studies, which may report falsely favourable or unfavourable prognoses, must therefore be viewed with caution. Table 1 outlines the key methodologic features of good prognostic studies and highlights those factors of particular importance for studies of prostate cancer.[18]

For any study of prognosis, it is important to identify patients at an early and uniform point in the course of their disease.[18] Because most "watchful waiting" studies of prostate cancer use data gathered retrospectively, it is difficult to ensure homogeneous inception cohorts. Some studies clearly fail this test. For example, one recent high-profile study[3] that reported surprisingly poor prognosis for initially untreated prostate cancer identified patients at a late stage in their disease (time of death), which ensured that slow-growing cancers would be substantially underrepresented.[19,20] Other studies included only incidental tumours found after simple prostatectomy,[9-11,15] and some included a significant proportion of patients with locally invasive and metastatic disease.[4,9,11,15] Finally, in several of the studies[1,3,6,14] cytology, rather than needle core biopsy, was used to diagnose and grade prostate cancer; this method may be associated with overdiagnosis.

Complete follow-up is important because members of an inception cohort who cannot be accounted for may bias the results.[18] In addition, because prostate cancer

Table 1: Key methodologic features of prognostic studies[18]

Assembly of inception cohort*

Description of referral pattern

Achievement of complete follow-up*

Use of objective outcome criteria*

Blind outcome assessment

Adjustment for extraneous prognostic factors*

*Of particular importance in studies of prostate cancer.

progresses slowly and outcome events are infrequent, reasonable sample sizes and follow-up periods of 10 to 15 years are necessary to estimate mortality rates accurately. Many of the published studies were small or had insufficiently long follow-up periods.[4,8,12,15]

> **KEY POINT**
> - In thinking about the natural history of prostate cancer, the time horizon should be 10 to 15 years, since follow-up periods of that duration are needed to estimate mortality rates accurately.

Defining outcome measures has been a particular problem in studies of prostate cancer. All-cause mortality rates in prostate cancer cohorts are of limited value because the death rates from prostate cancer and from other causes in this largely elderly patient group are of comparable magnitude.[21] Thus, differences in the distribution of coexisting disease in patient cohorts may dramatically affect overall mortality rates and render comparisons between cohorts meaningless. Death resulting directly from prostate cancer (cause-specific mortality) is probably a more objective endpoint but is still not without problems. It is not always possible to ascertain the cause of death in patients who had advanced prostate cancer. Published studies often have no explicit criteria for determining that death resulted from prostate cancer;[22] for those that do, the criteria differ from one study to another.[2,3]

When assessing outcome measures, it is important to control for prognostic factors that may have a significant influence on outcome.[18] For clinically localized prostate cancer, histologic grade is one such factor: the prognosis of poorly differentiated tumours is significantly different from that for well-differentiated tumours.[2] Differences in racial composition,[23,24] genetic differences controlling androgen metabolism[25] and susceptibility to metastasis,[26] smoking rates[27] and even physical activity[28] may also be important in the progression of prostate cancer. Although most studies report prognosis by tumour grade, no studies control for all of these more recently identified factors.

Finally, even the results of methodologically adequate studies may not be easily generalizable to patients in whom prostate cancer is diagnosed today. Most reported data, including those from the 3 prospective studies,[1,6,12] come from patients identified before 1987, when the era of testing for prostate-specific antigen (PSA) began.[29] Earlier cohorts may have presented with later-stage and higher-volume disease than grade-matched post-PSA cohorts. Thus, the prognosis of contemporary patients may be somewhat more favourable.

Gleason scoring system[31]	
Score is based on tumour differentiation and heterogenity Gleason score = sum of scores for 2 areas of a tumour Maximum value = 10	
Grade	Gleason score
1 (low)	2–4
2 (intermediate)	5–7
3 (high)	8–10

Results of the prognostic studies

Three studies[2,17,30] meet the minimum methodologic standards (Table 2). In these studies the single most important prognostic factor was histologic grade. In prostate cancer, grade is most commonly determined using the Gleason scoring system,[31] which is based on tumour differentiation and heterogeneity. The Gleason score is the sum of 2 scores of 1 to 5, each for a different area of the tumour. Patients with low-grade (grade 1, Gleason score 2–4) and intermediate-grade (grade 2, Gleason score 5–7) tumours appear to have the best prognosis, whereas the prognosis for patients with high-grade tumours (grade 3, Gleason score 8–10) is substantially worse.

Table 2 also shows 10-year cause-specific survival rates, stratified by tumour grade, from the 3 studies. Our best estimate for patients with untreated, clinically localized prostate cancer is that 9% to 66% will die from prostate cancer within 10 years, depending on histologic grade, the risk increasing with increasing tumour grade. Patients with low- and intermediate-grade tumours have a better prognosis (7% to 13% and 13% to 24% risk of death respectively), whereas patients with high-grade tumours have an unfavourable prognosis (46% to 66% risk of death). Thus, on the basis of tumour grade alone, the 65-year-old patient described in the case at the beginning of this article has a 13% to 24% probability of dying from prostate cancer within 10 years. However, his

Table 2: Characteristics of the 3 studies that meet the minimum methodologic standards for assessing the prognosis of clinically localized prostate cancer

Study	Strengths	Limitations	Tumour grade*; 10-yr prostate-cancer-specific survival rate, %		
			1	2	3
Lu-Yao and Yao[17] (n =18 238)†	Population-based with specific inclusion and exclusion criteria Large sample size Reports prostate-cancer-specific mortality rate Stratifies prognosis by stage, grade and comorbidity	Retrospective Uses data from an administrative database, which may have inaccuracies in grade, stage and treatment Mean follow-up 4 years	93	77	45
Albertsen et al[2] (n = 451)	Population-based with specific inclusion and exclusion criteria and detailed medical chart review Large sample size Mean follow-up 15.5 yr Reports prostate-cancer-specific mortality rate Stratifies prognosis by grade and comorbidity	Retrospective Definition of death from prostate cancer controversial Includes only patients aged 65 to 75 yr	91	76	54
Chodak et al[30] (n = 828)	Meta-analysis of 6 studies (2 prospective) Specific inclusion and exclusion criteria/Large sample size Mean follow-up 7 yr Reports prostate-cancer-specific mortality rate Stratifies prognosis by age, stage and grade	4 studies retrospective No detailed medical review	87	87	34

*1 = well differentiated, Gleason score 2–4; 2 = moderately differentiated, Gleason score 5–7; 3 = poorly differentiated, Gleason score 8–10.
†Data derived from the Surveillance, Epidemiology, and End Results (SEER) Program, which collects information on all cancer cases from 5 US states (Connecticut, Hawaii, New Mexico, Iowa and Utah) and 4 US metropolitan cities (San Francisco–Oakland, Detroit, Atlanta and Seattle).

true chance of dying from prostate cancer is a little lower, because there is a possibility that he will die from another cause within the next 10 years.

Another potentially important prognostic factor is tumour stage[32] (Table 3). Although this is a significant factor in influencing prostate-cancer-specific mortality when all stages of prostate cancer are considered (i.e., localized v. metastatic),[33] differences in stage within clinically localized tumours have not been shown to have independent prognostic value.[2,30] Clinically localized prostate cancer is defined as a tumour confined within the prostate with no evidence of regional or distant metastasis, as assessed by clinical, biochemical and radiographic tests. It is subdivided into tumours that are either nonpalpable by digital rectal examination (stage T1) or palpable but not extending outside the prostate (stage T2). After adjustment for histologic grade, no difference in prostate-cancer-specific survival has been observed for patients with stage T1 and T2 prostate cancer.[2,30]

A final issue to consider is the quality of life of patients living with prostate cancer. For patients treated conservatively, distant metastasis precedes death by a median period of 3 years.[22] The reduction in quality of life associated with advanced disease is substantial and may be as important as the prospect of death in evaluating prognosis.[34]

Table 3: Current methods of assessing stage of prostate cancer*

Stage	Criteria
T	*Refers to primary tumour; assessed by physical examination, imaging, endoscopy, biopsy and biochemical tests*
T1	Clinically inapparent tumour not palpable or visible by imaging
T1a	Tumour an incidental histologic finding in 5% or less of tissue resected (by TURP)
T1b	Tumour an incidental histologic finding in more than 5% of tissue resected (by TURP)
T1c	Tumour identified by needle biopsy (performed because of elevated PSA, for example)
T2	Tumour confined within the prostate
T2a	Tumour involves 1 lobe
T2b	Tumour involves 2 lobes
T3	Tumour extends through the prostatic capsule
T3a	Extracapsular extension (unilateral or bilateral)
T3b	Tumour invades seminal vesicle
T4	Tumour is fixed or invades adjacent structures other than seminal vesicles: bladder neck, external sphincter, rectum, levator muscles or pelvic wall
N	*Refers to regional lymph nodes; assessed by physical examination and imaging*
N0	No regional lymph node metastasis
N1	Regional lymph node metastasis
M	*Refers to distant metastasis; assessed by physical examination, imaging, skeletal studies and biochemical tests*
M0	No distant metastasis
M1	Distant metastasis
M1a	Nonregional lymph nodes
M1b	Bone(s)
M1c	Other site(s)

Note: TURP = transurethral resection of the prostate, PSA = prostate-specific antigen.
*Adapted from *TNM Classification of Malignant Tumours*, 5th ed. L.H. Sobin and C. Wittekind, editors. Copyright © 1997 Wiley-Liss Inc. Reprinted by permission of Wiley-Liss, Inc., a division of John Wiley & Sons, Inc.

Effects of age and comorbidity on prognosis

Age may affect prognosis in 2 ways: as a tumour factor and as a host factor. Tumour biology may be different in younger patients.[35] An inherited predisposition to prostate cancer may underlie both presentation at an early age and more aggressive tumour behaviour.[36] Age also affects the probability of dying from other diseases, which has a bearing on the question of whether a patient will live long enough to experience disease and death caused by prostate cancer.

To help illustrate this concept, we have used a model of life expectancy called the DEALE method (declining exponential approximation of life expectancy), in which patient-specific life expectancy is determined from the risks of competing causes of death, including the risk of death from a specific disease (e.g., prostate cancer), the risk of death from one or more coexisting diseases, and age-, sex- and race-related risk of death, which includes the risk of death from all other causes (Fig. 1).[37,38] It is important to recognize that this method involves assumptions, provides only approximate estimates of life expectancy and is used here only to illustrate the potential importance of age and comorbidity in the prognosis of prostate cancer.

Life expectancy for a man without cancer falls from approximately 22.3 years at age 55 to 9.1 years at age 75.[41] The difference in life expectancy for men with and without cancer provides an estimate of the average number of life years lost because of cancer in men who elect to be treated conservatively. Young men are clearly at highest risk of losing life

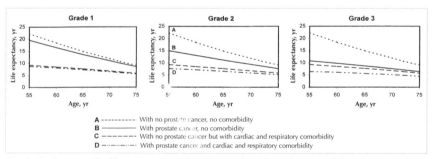

Fig. 1: Patient-specific life expectancy (PSLE) as a function of age and histologic grade of prostate cancer with and without coexisting cardiac and respiratory conditions, based on data from Albertsen and colleagues[2] and the DEALE method (declining exponential approximation of life expectancy).[37,38] PSLE = $1/(\Sigma\mu)$, where μ is the specific mortality rate for prostate cancer, the mortality rate(s) for coexisting conditions(s), and the age-, sex- and race-adjusted mortality rate (ASR). Mortality rates for coexisting cardiac and respiratory conditions are based on 10-year survival rates for patients with myocardial infarction[39] and mild chronic obstructive pulmonary disease,[40] where μ for a patient with myocardial infarction is 0.02039 and for a patient with mild chronic obstructive pulmonary disease is 0.04271. The μ_{ASR} values were obtained from Canadian Life Tables.[41]

years to cancer. For 55-year-old men, the loss of life expectancy because of cancer ranges from approximately 2 years for grade 1 disease to over 11 years for grade 3 disease. However, for men at age 75 the number of life years lost is much smaller, ranging from less than 1 year for grade 1 disease to 2 years for grade 3 disease. Clearly, young men with prostate cancer may lose many more potential life years to cancer than older men with disease of comparable grade and have a correspondingly higher risk of dying from, as opposed to with, their cancer.

> **KEY POINTS**
> - The most important tumour-specific variable for predicting prognosis is histologic grade.
> - The most important patient-specific factors in predicting prognosis are age and coexisting conditions.
> - The choice of therapy should take into account patient preferences for treatment-related outcomes, in addition to survival data.

The other host factor that affects the life expectancy of the patient described in the case is coexisting conditions, in this case, myocardial infarction and mild chronic obstructive pulmonary disease. The best empirical data we have about the effects of comorbidity on life expectancy in patients with prostate cancer are from Albertsen and colleagues.[2] In that study a validated comorbidity index was used to determine the prognostic importance of comorbidity in patients with prostate cancer. Comorbidity was a powerful predictor of overall survival — as powerful as tumour grade. This study illustrated 2 important points. First, comorbidity may pose an even higher risk of death than the cancer itself. Second, loss of life expectancy because of cancer is lower in men who have coexisting illnesses. Patients with a high burden of comorbidity are less likely to die from prostate cancer and, therefore, lose fewer years of life to prostate cancer, if they die early from another illness.

Fig. 1 illustrates the same point graphically by means of the DEALE method.[37,38,41] The number of life years lost because of cancer in a patient with coexisting conditions (in this case cardiac and respiratory conditions) is smaller than the number of life years lost because of cancer in a patient without such coexisting conditions. For our model, the specific mortality rates due to cardiac and respiratory disease are based on 10-year survival data for patients who had a myocardial infarction that was treated by thrombolysis and patients who had mild chronic obstructive pulmonary disease.[39,40] Our 65-year-old patient with grade 2 prostate cancer and cardiac and respiratory comorbidity would lose approximately 1.1 years of life expectancy because of the prostate cancer (Fig. 1, grade 2 tumour, line C minus line D), as opposed to about 3.7 years of life expectancy (line A minus line B) if he was as healthy as an average man of his age.

As a final caveat, when data such as these are applied to individual patients, it is important to keep in mind the fact that computing the number of life years lost because of disease does not translate into gains associated with treatment. It would be incorrect to infer, for example, that radical prostatectomy would result in an 11-year gain in life expectancy for a 55-year-old man with grade 3 disease. We still must rely on high-quality empirical evidence from controlled studies (e.g., randomized trials) to obtain reliable estimates of treatment benefit. Because there are no controlled data that reliably estimate the magnitude of treatment benefit associated with surgery and radiotherapy, life expectancy gains resulting from treatment are unknown. The number of life years lost because of cancer is best thought of as a potential upper bound on treatment benefit and probably a substantial overestimate of that benefit for any given patient, since disease recurrence and death occur in a substantial number of patients treated with surgery[42] and radiation.[43]

Watchful waiting versus definitive treatment

What about delaying surgery or radiotherapy until there is evidence of disease progression? As discussed above, our ability to predict which tumours will progress is related to grade and, to a lesser extent, stage for clinically localized prostate cancer. However, we do not yet have reliable clinical or laboratory tools to predict when the disease will progress for a specific patient. There are no data from randomized controlled trials that allow us to evaluate the strategy of delayed curative therapy. At present, observation strategies to monitor disease progression, such as PSA doubling times, are being investigated.[44] However, the role of this strategy remains uncertain, and it should not be considered equivalent to immediate curative therapy.

Even immediate curative therapy for clinically localized prostate cancer, as opposed to watchful waiting, remains controversial. The lack of high-quality evidence from prospective randomized trials comparing radical prostatectomy and radiotherapy with conservative management makes the task of recommending treatment particularly difficult. We must decide who should be treated with watchful waiting on the basis of relatively low-quality, complex data. Our 65-year-old patient presents a difficult treatment choice. We have seen that we must consider 3 factors: tumour grade, age and comorbidity. If our patient was a 75-year-old man with substantial comorbidity and low-grade disease, the decision would be more straightforward, and we would probably advise watchful waiting. If he was 55 and otherwise healthy, with high-grade disease, watchful waiting would likely not represent a good choice.

For this particular patient, the decision about which treatment to recommend will depend on what we consider a significant amount of life expectancy lost because of prostate cancer. In other words, is the potential gain in life expectancy of up to 1.1 years if this patient is treated clinically important, if we know that the actual gain will probably be less than that? Naimark and coworkers[45] have suggested that a life expectancy gain of 2 months is significant, given that it corresponds to risk reductions observed in clinical trials widely judged to have clinically significant outcomes. In general, a gain of 6 months has been considered significant by most analysts, a conclusion based on the gains for established treatment interventions such as smoking cessation (10.8 months) and cholecystectomy in asymptomatic diabetic patients (6.1 months).[46] Thus, a loss of 1.1 years from prostate cancer in a patient with substantial comorbidity can be considered clinically significant. However, it remains to be determined whether treatment will translate into a gain of 1.1 years.

Beyond age, grade and comorbidity, there is a fourth important factor: patient preference. Although this issue is not well understood, it is likely that individual patients value outcomes (e.g., sexual and urinary dysfunction) and risks of therapy differently. The morbidity associated with surgical and radiation therapy, including incontinence and impotence, is not trivial and is beginning to be better understood.[47] Some patients are extremely averse to risk and wish to avoid therapeutic complications at all costs. In highly risk-averse patients or those in whom preservation of sexual and urinary function is extremely important, watchful waiting could be considered a therapeutic option.

Decision-making for patients with localized prostate cancer is clearly not easy. From the available evidence, no concrete recommendation can be made, particularly for the patient described at the outset of this chapter. We know that we must consider age, histologic grade, comorbidity and personal preference. We have shown that the number of life years lost from prostate cancer in the setting of moderate comorbidity (cardiac and respiratory conditions) can be argued as clinically significant. However, the fact that we cannot guarantee an approximate gain of 1.1 years with treatment makes watchful waiting a reasonable alternative, and we will have to rely heavily on the patient's preference. Presenting the information in an objective, unbiased way, discussing his preferences about treatments and outcomes, and obtaining informed consent to the best of our ability is the most we can hope to achieve, given the present state of the evidence.

References

1. Johansson JE, Holmberg L, Johansson S, Bergstrom R, Adami HO. Fifteen-year survival in prostate cancer: a prospective, population-based study in Sweden. *JAMA* 1997;277:467-71.
2. Albertsen PC, Fryback DG, Storer BE, Kolon TF, Fine J. Long-term survival among

men with conservatively treated localized prostate cancer. *JAMA* 1995;274:626-31.
3. Aus G, Hugosson J, Norlen L. Long-term survival and mortality in prostate cancer treated with noncurative intent. *J Urol* 1995;154:460-5.
4. Bangma CH, Hop WCJ, Schroder FH. Serial prostate specific antigen measurements and progression in untreated confined (stages T0 to 3NxM0, grades 1 to 3) carcinoma of the prostate. *J Urol* 1995;154:1403-6.
5. Warner J, Whitmore WF Jr. Expectant management of clinically localized prostatic cancer. *J Urol* 1994;152:1761-5.
6. Adolfsson J, Carstensen J, Hedlund PO, Lowhagen T, Ronstrom L. Deferred treatment of clinically localized low grade prostate cancer: the experience from a prospective series at the Karolinska Hospital. *J Urol* 1994;152:1757-60.
7. Egawa S, Go M, Kuwao S, Shoji K, Uchida T, Koshiba K. Long-term impact of conservative management on localized prostate cancer. A twenty-year experience in Japan. *Urology* 1993;42:520-7.
8. Zbang G, Wasserman NF, Sidi AA, Reinberg Y, Reddy PK. Long-term followup results after expectant management of stage A1 prostatic cancer. *J Urol* 1991;146:99-103.
9. Stillwell TJ, Malek RS, Engen DE, Farrow GM. Incidental adenocarcinoma after open prostatic adenectomy. *J Urol* 1989;141:76-8.
10. Goodman CM, Busuttil A, Chisholm GD. Age, size and grade of tumour predict prognosis in incidentally diagnosed carcinoma of the prostate. *Br J Urol* 1988;62:576-80.
11. Handley R, Carr TW, Travis D, Powell H, Hall RR. Deferred treatment for prostate cancer. *Br J Urol* 1988;62:249-53.
12. George NJ. Natural history of localised prostatic cancer managed by conservative therapy alone. *Lancet* 1988;1:494-7.
13. Moskovitz B, Nitecki S, Levin DR. Cancer of the prostate: Is there a need for aggressive treatment? *Urol Int* 1987;42:49-52.
14. Larson A, Norlen BJ. Five-year follow-up of patients with localized prostatic carcinoma initially referred for expectant treatment [abstract]. *Scand J Urol Nephrol* 1985;19:30.
15. Cantrell BB, DeKlerk DP, Eggleston JC, Boitnott JK, Walsh PC. Pathological factors that influence prognosis in stage A prostatic cancer: the influence of extent versus grade. *J Urol* 1981;125:516-20.
16. Jones GW. Prospective, conservative management of localized prostate cancer. *Cancer* 1992;70:307-10.
17. Lu-Yao GL, Yao SL. Population-based study of long-term survival in patients with clinically localised prostate cancer. *Lancet* 1997;349:906-10.
18. Sackett DL, Haynes RB, Guyatt GH, Tugwell P. *Clinical epidemiology: a basic science for clinical medicine*. 2nd ed. Toronto: Little, Brown; 1991.
19. Abrahamsson PA, Adami HO, Taube A, Kim KM, Zelen M, Kulldorff M. Re: Long-term survival and mortality in prostate cancer treated with noncurative intent [letter]. *J Urol* 1996;155:296-8.
20. Chodak GW. What to expect from prostate cancer [editorial]. *J Urol* 1995;154:2132-3.
21. Lepor H, Kimball AW, Walsh PC. Cause-specific actuarial survival analysis: a useful method for reporting survival data in men with clinically localized carcinoma of the prostate. *J Urol* 1989;141:82-4.
22. Chodak GW, Vogelzang NJ, Caplan RJ, Soloway MS, Smith JA. Independent prognostic factors in patients with metastatic (stage D2) prostate cancer. *JAMA*

1991;265:618-21.
23. Ross RK, Coetzee GA, Reichardt J, Skinner E, Henderson BE. Does the racial–ethnic variation in prostate cancer risk have a hormonal basis? *Cancer* 1995;75:1780.
24. Optenberg SA, Thompson IM, Friedrichs P, Wojcik B, Stein CR, Kramer B. Race, treatment, and long-term survival from prostate cancer in an equal-access medical care delivery system. *JAMA* 1995;274:1599-605.
25. Gann PH, Hennekens CH, Ma J, Longcope C, Stampfer MJ. Prospective study of sex hormone levels and risk of prostate cancer. *J Natl Cancer Inst* 1996;88:1118-26.
26. Dong JT, Lamb PW, Rinker-Schaeffer CW, Vukanovic J, Ichikawa T, Isaacs JT, et al. KAI1, a metastasis suppressor gene for prostate cancer on human chromosome 11p11.2. *Science* 1995;268:884-6.
27. Rodriguez C, Tatham LM, Thun MJ, Calle EE, Heath CW. Smoking and fatal prostate cancer in a large cohort of adult men. *Am J Epidemiol* 1997;145:466-75.
28. Lee IM, Paffenbarger RS, Hsieh CC. Physical activity and risk of prostatic cancer among college alumni. *Am J Epidemiol* 1992;135:169-79.
29. Stamey TA, Yang N, Hay R, McNeal JE, Freiha FS, Redwine E. Prostate-specific antigen as a serum marker for adenocarcinoma of the prostate. *N Engl J Med* 1987;317:909-15.
30. Chodak GW, Thisted RA, Gerber GS, Johansson JE, Adolfsson J, Jones GW, et al. Results of conservative management of clinically localized prostate cancer. *N Engl J Med* 1994;330:242-8.
31. Gleason DF, Mellinger GT. Prediction of prognosis for prostatic adenocarcinoma by combined histological grading and clinical staging. *J Urol* 1974;111(1):58-64.
32. Urological tumours. In: Sobin LH, Wittekind C, editors. *TNM classification of malignant tumours*. 5th ed. New York: Wiley-Liss, Inc; 1997. p. 170-3.
33. Mettlin C, Jones GW, Murphy GP. Trends in prostate cancer care in United States, 1974-1990: observations from the patient care evaluation studies of the American College of Surgeons Commission on Cancer. *CA Cancer J Clin* 1993;43:83-91.
34. Da Silva FC. Quality of life in prostatic cancer patients. *Cancer* 1993;72:3803-6.
35. Gronberg H, Damber JE, Jonsson H, Lenner P. Patient age as a prognostic factor in prostate cancer. *J Urol* 1994;152:892-5.
36. Carter BS, Beaty TH, Steinberg GD, Childs B, Walsh PC. Mendelian inheritance of familial prostate cancer. *Proc Natl Acad Sci U S A* 1992;89:3367-71.
37. Beck JR, Kassirer JP, Pauker SG. A convenient approximation of life expectancy: 1. Validation of the method. *Am J Med* 1982;73:883-8.
38. Beck JR, Pauker SG, Gotlieb JE, Klein K, Kassirer JP. A convenient approximation of life expectancy (the "DEALE"): 2. Use in medical decision-making. *Am J Med* 1982;73:889-97.
39. Mark DB, Hlatky MA, Califf RM, Naylor CD, Lee KL, Armstrong PW, et al. Cost effectiveness of thrombolytic therapy with tissue plasminogen activator as compared with streptokinase for acute myocardial infarction. *N Engl J Med* 1995;332:1418-24.
40. Burrows B, Bloom JW, Traver GA, Cline MG. The course and prognosis of different forms of chronic airways obstruction in a sample from the general population. *N Engl J Med* 1987;317:1309-14.
41. Statistics Canada. Life tables: Canada and provinces. *Health Rep* 1990;2:17.
42. Gerber GS, Thisted RA, Scardino PT, Frohmuller HG, Schroeder FH, Paulson DF, et al. Results of radical prostatectomy in men with clinically localized prostate cancer.

JAMA 1996;276:615-9.
43. Duncan W, Warde P, Catton CN, Munro AJ, Lakier R, Gadaila T, et al. Carcinoma of the prostate: results of radical radiotherapy (1970–1985). *Int J Radiat Oncol Biol Phys* 1993;26:203-10.
44. Nam RK, Klotz LH, Jewett MAS, Danjoux C, Trachtenberg J. Prostate specific antigen velocity as a measure of the natural history of prostate cancer: defining a "rapid riser" subset. *Br J Urol* 1998;81:100-4.
45. Naimark D, Naglie G, Detsky AS. The meaning of life expectancy: What is clinically significant gain? *J Gen Intern Med* 1994;9:702-7.
46. Krahn MD, Naglie G, Naimark D, Redelmeier DA, Detsky AS. Primer on medical decision analysis: Part 4. Analyzing the model and interpreting the results. *Med Decis Making* 1997;17:142-51.
47. Lim AJ, Brandon AH, Fiedler J, Brickman AL, Boyer CI, Raub WA Jr, et al. Quality of life: radical prostatectomy versus radiation therapy for prostate cancer. *J Urol* 1995;154:1420-5.

3

Individual risk factors

Richard P. Gallagher, MA; Neil E. Fleshner, MD, MPH

> A 42-year-old lawyer makes an appointment to see his family physician. His father (age 67) has just been diagnosed with metastatic prostate cancer. The patient has no significant medical history and has not seen a doctor since he had a vasectomy 7 years ago. He is an admitted junk-food addict, has a sedentary lifestyle and is moderately overweight. Palpation reveals no abnormalities of the prostate. The patient asks the physician's advice about reducing his risk of prostate cancer.

Rising incidence rates and increased public awareness of prostate cancer have created an explosion of scientific interest in the epidemiology of this disease.[1] Although a number of studies are shedding light on risk factors, the data are not firm enough to support widescale primary prevention trials. Nevertheless, the importance of several factors is becoming clear (Fig. 1).

National and ethnic differences

In Canada, the incidence rates for prostate cancer are among the highest in the world, although they are still below those in the United States and Sweden.[1,2] The highest incidence rates occur among black American men, for whom the age-standardized rates are 50% to 60% higher than those for white American men.[2] The lowest rates of prostate cancer are typically found in Asian countries; the rates in China are only 4% of those in Canada.[3]

KEY POINTS
- Prostate cancer incidence and mortality rates vary from country to country: those in Western nations (including Canada) are among the highest; those in Asian countries (including China and Japan) are low.
- Populations migrating from low- to high-risk areas experience increased rates of prostate cancer, which suggests that environment plays an important role in disease causation.

Although variations in case-finding strategies may provide a partial explanation, these differences are much too pronounced to be artifacts due entirely to ascertainment procedures.

Studies of migrating populations are often useful in determining the relative contributions of genetics and environment to disease causation. Among Asian men who have immigrated to North America, for example, prostate cancer incidence rates remain low. Within long-standing Chinese and Japanese communities in North America, these rates, although much higher than in Asia, are only about half those for white men living in the same areas.[2] Although these racial differences suggest a genetic component to disease causation, cultural practices, such as dietary habits, may also explain the variations. Furthermore, the fact that incidence rates increase significantly in groups who immigrate to North America indicates that lifestyle factors play a major role in the etiology of the disease.

Family history and genetic predisposition

Apart from age, the most consistent risk factor for prostate cancer found to

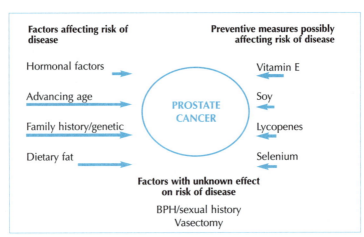

Fig. 1: Common risk factors and preventive factors for prostate cancer. Arrow length is proportional to the degree of supporting evidence. Factors listed to the left and right of the circle indicate risks and preventive factors, respectively. For benign prostatic hyperplasia (BPH) or sexual history and vasectomy, there is very little evidence supporting the association.

date is the occurrence of the disease in a close relative.[4] Having a first-degree relative (i.e., a father, son or brother) with prostate cancer increases the risk of the disease by about 2 to 2.5 times among black, white and Asian men in North America.[4–7] If 2 or more first-degree relatives have prostate cancer, the risk increases by more than 4 times among white and Asian men and by perhaps as much as 10 times among black North American men.[6] A recent Canadian study[8] found that the risk associated with having 1 or more relatives with the disease was midway between the risk associated with having 1 relative affected and that of having 2 or more relatives affected. The risk associated with having a first-degree relative with the disease may be even higher if that relative's diagnosis is made before age 65, although this is still to be confirmed.[7]

> **KEY POINTS**
> - Apart from age, family history is the most consistent risk factor for prostate cancer.
> - Risk escalates as the number of first-degree relatives affected increases, and risk is higher among those with relatives in whom the disease was detected at an early age.
> - Epidemiologic analysis suggests that there may be one or more genes for familial prostate cancer, but this has yet to be confirmed.

Elevation of risk of prostate cancer among relatives may be attributed to genetic predisposition, shared exposures or bias. Genetic factors appear to be partly responsible for familial clustering, and a recent segregation analysis[9] suggested that an autosomal dominant gene might be responsible. The proposed model suggests that about 0.6% of white men inherit a mutated allele of one or more predisposing genes, which confers a lifetime risk of prostate cancer for these men of about 88%, as opposed to about 5% for men without the mutated allele. The model suggests a relative risk of about 1.6 for men whose fathers have prostate cancer compared with men whose fathers do not have the disease; this estimate is similar to, although slightly lower than, what has been seen in recent studies.[4,6]

Clustering of prostate cancer has also been reported in more distant relative pairs, such as grandfather–grandson, uncle–nephew, first cousins and second cousins.[10] It is unlikely that this effect is due to detection bias or shared environmental factors.

A number of groups have provided evidence of a "prostate cancer gene," *HPC1*, on the short arm of chromosome 1.[11,12] A great deal more work is needed to identify the specific mutated locus within this region, which contains 20 million base pairs, and to determine the function of the gene. The fact that at least one group studying large numbers of high-risk families[13] has not confirmed the importance of *HPC1* suggests that this marker is not the only gene predisposing men to familial prostate cancer. Other studies have pointed to different candidates, including several genes on the X chromosome,[14] such as the androgen receptor gene[15] and the vitamin D receptor gene.[16]

Diet

Descriptive data suggest that diet plays a major role in prostate cancer. Internationally, the incidence of prostate cancer is highly correlated with that of colon, breast and endometrial cancers, which are thought to be related to diet.[17] The rate of death from prostate cancer for Japanese men increases when they immigrate to North America, and dietary changes are thought to be a significant factor in these increases.[18]

Dietary fat

Data from analytic studies suggest a positive relation between high fat consumption and prostate cancer[19–34] (Appendix 1). Although some of the early studies[19,21,22] revealed no association, dietary assessment became more sophisticated in later investigations. The first study to include both large numbers of cases and controls and a dietary assessment questionnaire that identified the majority (85%) of normal intake[24] showed that prostate cancer incidence increased with consumption of saturated fat in most of the ethnic groups studied.

The association between dietary fat and aggressiveness of the cancer raises the possibility that fat primarily affects disease progression within established tumours. A recent study[35] carried out in mice with established transplanted human prostate tumours and raised on a diet with 40% of calories from fat suggested that reduction to 20% of calories from fat slowed tumour growth velocity relative to mice maintained on the high-fat diet. If these observations are confirmed, reducing dietary fat may reduce the risk of prostate cancer, even relatively late in life.

Micronutrients

Many studies[20–24,28,29,32,34,36–40] have reported on the putative relation between vitamin A or β-carotene intake and prostate cancer (Appendix 2). These compounds are potent antioxidants and may exert a protective effect against epithelial tumours. Unfortunately, there is no consistent evidence of protection from prostate cancer and, in fact, several studies[24,39] have suggested that these nutrients increase the risk of this disease.

Vitamin E

Although there is relatively little information on the effect of vitamin E, or α-tocopherol (its most common form), some recent findings[34,41] suggest that it may reduce the risk of prostate cancer. However, other results[37,39] have not been convincing, and more work is necessary to assess this potential association.

Lycopene and tomato products

Consumption of tomatoes and tomato-based products may reduce the risk of prostate cancer.[27,39] Researchers have concluded that lycopene, a potent antioxidant found in tomatoes, may be responsible. Recent evidence also indicates that levels of lycopene in the prostate are at high enough concentrations to be equivalent to those that are biologically active in laboratory studies.[42] More research is needed to clarify the role of lycopene in prostate cancer.

> **KEY POINTS**
> - A diet high in fat has been associated with an increased risk of prostate cancer.
> - Dietary fat may be particularly associated with aggressive cancers, which suggests a role in disease progression.
> - Vitamin E and selenium may reduce the incidence of prostate cancer.
> - The potential preventive properties of soy products and lycopenes are being investigated.

Selenium

Glutathione peroxidase, an enzyme that protects cells from oxidative damage, is selenium dependent,[43] and several epidemiologic studies have confirmed an inverse association between selenium intake and various human cancers, including prostate cancer.[43] Recently, the efficacy of 200 µg/day of selenomethionine in a placebo-controlled intervention study of 1312 patients with non-melanoma skin cancer was reported.[44] After 8269 patient-years of follow-up, there was a 3- to 4-fold lower incidence of prostate cancer among those who received the selenium (relative risk 0.29, $p < 0.001$). No toxic effects of selenium were observed. Although the incidence of prostate cancer was not an intended outcome variable in this study, these highly significant findings call for further investigation.

Soy products

The incidence of prostate cancer is significantly lower in Asia than in North America,[2] and some of this difference is thought to be due to diet. A recent investigation of serum levels of 2 isoflavones, daidizein and genistein, in normal Japanese and Finnish men revealed substantially higher concentrations in the Japanese men.[45] Isoflavones are phytochemicals that possess a wide range of anticancer properties. Genistein, which occurs in lentils and soy products such as tofu, inhibits the growth of androgen-dependent and androgen-independent prostate cancer cells in culture.[46]

To date only one study[26] of tofu consumption has shown a protective effect in terms of prostate cancer risk. Another study[27] demonstrated that lentils and beans, which are known to contain isoflavones, have a protective effect. Currently, there is insufficient evidence to recommend an increase in consumption of isoflavinoids, but further research may well identify a chemopreventive effect for prostate cancer.

Body mass and physical activity

Case–control studies[47–50] have suggested that men with high body mass and those who are obese as adults have an increased risk of prostate cancer; however, others[27,29,32] have failed to confirm this association. Level of physical activity has been found to be inversely associated with risk,[31,51] but the data are inconsistent with other studies showing an association or a positive relation.[29,32,48] This association may have to be examined in young men, in whom physical activity is known to affect hormonal profiles.[52]

Vasectomy

Evidence for a relation between prostate cancer and vasectomy is inconclusive. Currently, the consensus appears to be that even if vasectomy is a risk factor for prostate cancer, it is a weak one, and its effect is not strong enough to influence public health policy regarding vasectomy.[53]

Hormonal and sexual factors

Sex hormones are probably related to the development of prostate cancer for several reasons: the prostate gland is androgen dependent,[54] prostate cancer does not occur in eunuchs,[55] administration of male sex hormones can induce prostate cancer in animal models,[54] and castration induces programmed cell death — apoptosis — in prostate cancer cells.[56]

A recent study of normal, older, black, white and Asian men[57] — groups known to be at high, medium and low risk for prostate cancer respectively — showed that after adjustment for age and body mass, the levels of total and bioavailable testosterone were highest in Asian men, intermediate in white men and lowest in black men. However, the ratio of dihydrotestosterone to testosterone was the reverse (i.e., highest in black men, intermediate in white men and lowest in Asian men). Also, sex hormone binding globulin (SHBG) levels were higher in men reporting one or more first-degree relatives with prostate cancer. A prospective cohort study[58] revealed that high plasma levels of testosterone before diagnosis were associated with increased risk of prostate cancer, and an inverse trend was seen with levels of SHBG. Thus, data in this area are contradictory, and further study is necessary.

Several studies[59,60] have suggested that subjects with shorter polymorphic CAG repeat sequences in the androgen receptor gene are at higher risk for prostate cancer than those with longer sequences. This finding suggests that male sex hormone regulation is critical in the development of prostate cancer, which might account for the lower risk of prostate cancer in Asian men.

Because sex hormone levels decline with age,[57] investigators are beginning to evaluate the hormonal profiles of young men, reasoning that the etiologically relevant period may be at a much younger age than the age at which the cancer develops. Serum

> **KEY POINTS**
> - Physical activity and obesity have not been consistently associated with prostate cancer.
> - Evidence does not support the suggestion that vasectomy is a risk factor.
> - Hormonal milieu is important in the development of prostate cancer; however, additional work is needed to determine which steroidal metabolites are important and at what ages.

testosterone levels in college-aged black men have been found to be 15% higher, and free testosterone levels 13% higher, than in their white counterparts.[61] These differences are substantially greater than in older black, white and Asian men. In another study that included young Japanese men as well as black and white American men,[62] the expected low levels of testosterone in the Japanese men were not found. However, there was indirect evidence of reduced 5 α-reductase activity in the Japanese men, which may account for the low rate of clinically evident prostate cancer in Japan.

Because diet and levels of physical activity can affect male serum hormone levels,[63] more research is needed on these factors, particularly among young men of various ethnic groups. It would also be useful to compare dietary patterns and serum hormone levels in young men whose fathers or grandfathers have prostate cancer with those of young men without a family history of the disease.

Sexual history

Studies of sexual history in men with and without prostate cancer have not, by and large, revealed consistent differences. Several investigations[64,65] have suggested that men with prostate cancer were sexually active earlier and had more partners than the control group, but other evidence appears to indicate the opposite.[66] History of sexual activity seems to be open to substantial misclassification, and because the information gathered is impossible to validate, it is difficult to imagine that this will be a fruitful area for future study.

Benign prostatic hyperplasia

Benign prostatic hyperplasia (BPH) is common in older men; it varies considerably in onset and severity and is difficult to study because of the lack of standardized pathologic criteria for its diagnosis. Several epidemiologic investigations have been conducted to evaluate whether men with BPH are at higher risk for prostate cancer. One of these studies[67] identified a higher risk of prostate cancer among those with BPH, but another,[68] a follow-up comparison of a cohort of patients who underwent subtotal prostatectomy for BPH with a group of other surgical patients, found no increase in risk.

Historically, men with symptomatic BPH have undergone transurethral prostate surgery, and in 10% of cases cancer has been discovered incidentally. Given this detection bias, only death from prostate cancer could serve as an adequate endpoint. Fortunately, the detailed embryologic and anatomic studies of McNeal[69] have shed some light on this issue. Benign prostate disease is restricted to the transition zone compartment of the prostate gland. Conversely, prostate cancer originates principally in the peripheral zone compartment. This critical difference in disease ontogeny suggests that a causal relation between these 2 conditions is unlikely.

Occupational exposure

The role of occupational exposure in the etiology of prostate cancer has been explored. Several cohort investigations have found an elevated risk among workers exposed to cadmium,[70] although other studies,[71-73] including expanded analyses[72,73] for one of the occupational groups for which a positive association had previously been found, have shown no increased risk.

Although potential biologic mechanisms for carcinogenesis have been suggested,[72] it seems unlikely that cadmium exposure alone could explain much of the current prevalence of prostate cancer. Using sound data on exposure, Aronson and coworkers[74] found elevated risks among those employed in the water-transport and aircraft manufacturing industries. Other groups at elevated risk include metal product fabricators, structural metal erectors and railway transport workers. The difficulty with these associations is that no dose–response relation is seen, with the possible exception of exposure to aluminum dust and to liquid fuel combustion products.

Farming and agricultural work have been associated with elevated mortality rate from prostate cancer in several studies;[75,76] however, others have failed to validate these observations.[74,77] Recent investigations have revealed high incidence of and mortality rates from cancer among airline pilots[78] and chemical workers exposed to perfluorooctanoic acid.[79] However, with the possible exception of perfluorooctanoic acid, even if the higher rates observed are "real," primary prevention programs in the workplace would be difficult to implement because specific carcinogens have not been identified.

Conclusion

The aging of the Canadian population and the longer life expectancy of men have made prostate cancer a major public health issue. Thus, the research community must intensify efforts to elucidate the etiology of this disease in the expectation that many of the risk factors identified will be modifiable. Several research areas look promising:
- Studies of the cascade of mutations that mark the transformation of normal prostatic tissue to frank carcinoma may help to identify specific loci of action for carcinogens in sporadic prostate cancer.
- Studies aimed at isolating germline mutations that predispose to familial prostate cancer will help identify men at high risk long before the disease occurs.
- Dietary studies with emphasis on the early years of life, coupled with investigation of physical activity levels and serum hormone levels, might reveal more about early events critical in the occurrence of the disease.
- Studies of hormone profiles in young men of various ethnic groups, particularly in families with a strong history of prostate cancer, could identify early hormonal anomalies leading to higher risk later in life.

The patient described in the case at the beginning of this article is at elevated risk for prostate cancer. The main risk relates to his father's disease, but other factors, in order of diminishing significance, are his high-fat diet and his sedentary lifestyle. In terms of clinical recommendations, there are as yet no evidence-based guidelines. However, in terms of overall health, the patient would be wise to decrease his fat intake and begin an exercise program. Consumption of vitamin E and tofu are unlikely to cause harm and may provide beneficial effects. Although there are no firm guidelines regarding screening, the American Urological Association recommends that digital rectal examination and testing for prostate-specific antigen begin at age 40.[80]

References

1. National Cancer Institute of Canada. *Canadian cancer statistics 1998.* Toronto: The Institute; 1998. p. 28.
2. Parkin DM, Muir CS, Whelan SL, Gao YT, Ferlay J, Powell J. *Cancer incidence in five continents.* Vol 6. Lyon, France: International Agency for Research on Cancer; 1992. Sci publ 120.
3. Whittemore AS. Colorectal cancer incidence among Chinese in North America and the People's Republic of China: variation with sex, age and anatomical site. *Int J Epidemiol* 1989;18:563-8.
4. Steinberg GD, Carter BS, Beaty TH, Childs B, Walsh PC. Family history and the risk of prostate cancer. *Prostate* 1990;17:337-47.

5. Hayes R, Liff J, Pottern L, Greenberg R, Schoenberg J, Schwartz A, et al. Prostate cancer risk in U.S. blacks and whites with a family history of cancer. *Int J Cancer* 1995;60:361-4.
6. Whittemore AS, Wu A, Kolonel L, John E, Gallagher RP, Howe G, et al. Family history and prostate cancer risk in black, white, and Asian men in the United States and Canada. *Am J Epidemiol* 1995;141:732-40.
7. Lesko SM, Rosenberg L, Shapiro S. Family history and prostate cancer risk. *Am J Epidemiol* 1996;144:1041-7.
8. Ghadirian P, Howe GR, Hislop TG, Maisonneuve P. Family history of prostate cancer: a multi-centre case–control study in Canada. *Int J Cancer* 1997;70:679-81.
9. Carter BS, Beaty TH, Steinberg G, Childs B, Walsh PC. Mendelian inheritance of familial prostate cancer. *Proc Natl Acad Sci U S A* 1992;89:3367-71.
10. Cannon-Albright L, Thomas A, Goldgar GE, Gholami K, Rowe K, Jacobsen M, et al. Familiality of prostate cancer in Utah. *Cancer Res* 1994;54:2378-85.
11. Smith JR, Freije D, Carpten JD, Gronberg H, Xu J, Isaacs SD, et al. Major susceptibility locus for prostate cancer on chromosome 1 suggested by genome-wide search. *Science* 1996;274:1371-4.
12. Cooney KA, McCarthy JD, Lange E, Huang L, Miesfield S, Montie J, et al. Prostate cancer susceptibility locus on chromosome 1q: a confirmatory study. *J Natl Cancer Inst* 1997;89:955-9.
13. McIndoe RA, Stanford JL, Gibbs M, Jarvik GP, Brandzel S, Neal CL, et al. Linkage analysis of 49 high-risk families does not support a common familial prostate cancer-susceptibility gene at 1q24–25. *Am J Hum Genet* 1997;61:347-55.
14. Monroe KR, Yu MC, Kolonel LN, Coetze GA, Wilkens L, Ross RK, et al. Evidence of an X-linked or recessive genetic component to prostate cancer risk. *Nat Med* 1995;1:827-9.
15. Ingles SA, Ross RK, Yu M, Irvine RA, LaPera G, Haile RW, et al. Association of prostate cancer risk with genetic polymorphisms in vitamin D receptor and androgen receptor. *J Natl Cancer Inst* 1997;89:166-70.
16. Feldman D. Androgen and vitamin D receptor gene polymorphisms: the long and short of prostate cancer risk. *J Natl Cancer Inst* 1997;89:109-11.
17. Hunter DJ, Willett WC. Diet, body size and breast cancer. *Epidemiol Rev* 1993;15:110-32.
18. Haenszel W, Kurihara M. Studies of Japanese migrants. I. Mortality from cancer and other diseases among Japanese in the United States. *J Natl Cancer Inst* 1968;40:43-68.
19. Hirayama T. *Epidemiology of prostate cancer with special reference to the role of diet.* Bethesda: National Cancer Institute; 1979. p. 149-55. Monogr 53.
20. Graham S, Haughey B, Marshall J, Priore R, Byers T, Rzepka T, et al. Diet in the epidemiology of carcinoma of the prostate gland. *J Natl Cancer Inst* 1983;70:687-92.
21. Ohno Y, Yoshida O, Oishi K, Okada K, Yamabe H, Schroeder FH. Dietary beta-carotene and cancer of the prostate: a case–control study in Kyoto, Japan. *Cancer Res* 1988;48:1331-6.
22. Kaul L, Heshmet M, Kovi J, Jackson MA, Jackson AG, Jones GW, et al. The role of diet in prostate cancer. *Nutr Cancer* 1987;9:123-8.
23. Ross RK, Shimuzu H, Paganini-Hill A, Honda G, Henderson BE. Case–control study of prostate cancer in blacks and whites in southern California. *J Natl Cancer Inst* 1987;78:869-74.

24. Kolonel LN, Yoshizawa CN, Hanken JH. Diet and prostatic cancer: a case–control study in Hawaii. *Am J Epidemiol* 1988;127:999-1012.
25. Mettlin C, Selenkas S, Natarajan N, Huben R. Beta-carotene and animal fats and their relationship to prostate cancer risk, a case–control study. *Cancer* 1989;64:605-12.
26. Severson RK, Nomura A, Grove JS, Stemmermann GN. A prospective study of demographics, diet and prostate cancer among men of Japanese ancestry in Hawaii. *Cancer Res* 1989;49:1857-60.
27. Mills PK, Beeson L, Phillips R, Fraser GE. Cohort study of diet, lifestyle and prostate cancer in Adventist men. *Cancer* 1989;64:598-604.
28. Hsing AW, McLaughlin JK, Schuman LM, Bjelke E, Gridley G, Wacholder S, et al. Diet, tobacco use, and fatal prostate cancer: results from the Lutheran Brotherhood cohort study. *Cancer Res* 1990;50:6836-40.
29. West D, Slattery ML, Robison LM, French TK, Mahoney AW. Adult dietary intake and prostate cancer in Utah: a case–control study with special emphasis on aggressive tumors. *Cancer Causes Control* 1991;2:85-94.
30. Giovannucci E, Rimm E, Colditz G, Stampfer MJ, Ascherio A, Chute C, et al. A prospective study of dietary fat and risk of prostate cancer. *J Natl Cancer Inst* 1993;85:1571-9.
31. Andersson SO, Baron J, Wolk A, Lindgren C, Bergstrom R, Adami HO. Early life risk factors for prostate cancer: a population-based case–control study in Sweden. *Cancer Epidemiol Biomarkers Prev* 1995;4:187-92.
32. Whittemore AS, Kolonel LN, Wu AH, John E, Gallagher RP, Howe GR, et al. Prostate cancer in relation to diet, physical activity and body size in blacks, whites and Asians in the United States and Canada. *J Natl Cancer Inst* 1995;87:652-61.
33. Rohan T, Howe G, Burch JD, Jain M. Dietary factors and risk of prostate cancer: a case–control study in Ontario, Canada. *Cancer Causes Control* 1995;6:145-54.
34. Vlajinac HD, Marinkovic JM, Ilic MD, Kovec NI. Diet and prostate cancer: a case–control study. *Eur J Cancer* 1997;33:101-7.
35. Wang Y, Corr JG, Thaler HT, Tao Y, Fair WR, Heston WD. Decreased growth of established human prostate LNCaP tumors in nude mice fed a low-fat diet. *J Natl Cancer Inst* 1995;87:1456-62.
36. Paganini-Hill A, Chao A, Ross RK, Henderson BE. Vitamin A, beta-carotene, and risk of cancer: a prospective study. *J Natl Cancer Inst* 1987;79:443-8.
37. Hayes R, Bogdanovicz J, Schroeder F, DeBruijn A, Raatgever J, van der Maas P, et al. Serum retinol and prostate cancer. *Cancer* 1988;62:2021-6.
38. Reichman M, Hayes R, Ziegler R, Schatzkin A, Taylor P, Kahle L, et al. Serum vitamin A and subsequent development of prostate cancer in the First National Health and Nutrition Examination Survey epidemiologic follow-up study. *Cancer Res* 1990;50:2311-5.
39. Giovannucci E, Ascherio A, Rimm E, Stampfer M, Colditz G, Willett W. Intake of carotenoid and retinol in relation to risk of prostate cancer. *J Natl Cancer Inst* 1995;87:1767-76.
40. Daviglus M, Dyer A, Persky V, Chavez N, Drum M, Goldberg J, et al. Dietary beta-carotene, vitamin C, and risk of prostate cancer: results from the Western Electric study. *Epidemiology* 1996;7:472-7.
41. Alpha-tocopherol Beta-carotene Cancer Prevention Study Group. The effect of vitamin E and beta-carotene on the incidence of lung cancer and other cancers in male smokers. *N Engl J Med* 1994;330:1029-35.

42. Clinton SK, Emenhiser C, Schwartz SJ, Bostwick DG, Williams AW, Moore BJ, et al. Cis-trans lycopene isomers, carotenoids, and retinol in the human prostate. *Cancer Epidemiol Biomarkers Prev* 1996;5:823-33.
43. El-Barjoumi K. The role of selenium in cancer prevention. In: DeVita VT, Hellman S, Rosenberg S, editors. *Cancer prevention*. Philadelphia: JB Lippincott; 1991. p. 1-15.
44. Clark LC, Combs GR Jr, Turnbull BW, Slate EH, Chalker DK, Chow J, et al. Effects of selenium supplementation for cancer prevention in patients with carcinoma of the skin. *JAMA* 1996;267:1957-63.
45. Aldercreutz H, Markannen H, Watanabe S. Plasma concentrations of phyto-estrogens in Japanese men. *Lancet* 1993;342:1209-10.
46. Peterson G, Barnes S. Genistein and biochanin A inhibit the growth of human prostate cancer cells but not epidermal growth factor receptor tyrosine autophosphorylation. *Prostate* 1993;22:335-45.
47. Snowdon D, Phillips R, Choi W. Diet obesity and risk of fatal prostate cancer. *Am J Epidemiol* 1984;120:244-50.
48. Cerhan JR, Torner J, Lynch CF, Rubenstein LM, Lemke JH, Cohen MB, et al. Association of smoking, body mass, and physical activity with risk of prostate cancer in the Iowa 65+ rural health study (United States). *Cancer Causes Control* 1997;8:229-38.
49. Talamini R, La Veechra C, DiCarli A. Nutrition, social factors and prostate cancer in a northern Italian population. *Br J Cancer* 1986;53:817-21.
50. Giovanucci E, Rimm E, Stampfer M, Colditz G, Willett W. Height, body weight and risk of prostate cancer. *Cancer Epidemiol Biomarkers Prev* 1997;6:557-63.
51. Thune I, Lund E. Physical activity and the risk of prostate and testicular cancer; a cohort study of 53 000 Norwegian men. *Cancer Causes Control* 1994;5:549-56.
52. Wheeler G, Wall S, Belcastro N, Cumming D. Reduced serum testosterone and prolactin levels in male distance runners. *JAMA* 1984;252:514-6.
53. Guess HA. Is vasectomy a risk factor for prostate cancer? *Eur J Cancer* 1993;29A:1055-60.
54. Noble RL. The development of prostatic adenocarcinoma in Nb rat following prolonged sex hormone administration. *Cancer Res* 1977;37:1929-33.
55. Ross R, Paganini-Hill A, Henderson B. The etiology of prostate cancer: What does the epidemiology suggest? *Prostate* 1983;4:333-44.
56. Catalona W. Management of cancer of the prostate. *N Engl J Med* 1994;331:996-1004.
57. Wu A, Whittemore A, Kolonel L, John E, Gallagher RP, West D, et al. Serum androgens and sex hormone-binding globulins in relation to lifestyle factors in older African-American, white and Asian men in the United States and Canada. *Cancer Epidemiol Biomarkers Prev* 1995;4:735-41.
58. Gann PH, Hennekens CH, Ma J, Longcope C, Stampfer MJ. Prospective study of sex hormone levels and risk of prostate cancer. *J Natl Cancer Inst* 1996;88:1118-26.
59. Giovannucci E, Stampfer MJ, Krithivas K, Brufsky A, Talcott J, Hennekens CH, et al. The CAG repeat within androgen receptor gene and its relationship to prostate cancer. *Proc Natl Acad Sci U S A* 1997;94:3320-3.
60. Stanford JL, Just JJ, Gibbs M, Wicklund KG, Neal CL, Blumenstein BA, et al. Polymorphic repeats in the androgen receptor gene: molecular marker of prostate cancer risk. *Cancer Res* 1997;57:1194-8.
61. Ross R, Bernstein L, Judd H, Hamische R, Pike M, Henderson B. Serum testosterone levels in healthy black and white men. *J Natl Cancer Inst* 1986;76:45-8.
62. Ross R, Bernstein L, Lobo R, Shimuzu H, Stanczyk F, Pike M, et al. 5-Alpha-

reductase activity and risk of prostate cancer among Japanese and US white and black males. *Lancet* 1992;339:887-9.
63. Wheeler G, Wall S, Belcastro N, Cumming D. Reduced serum testosterone and prolactin levels in male distance runners. *JAMA* 1984;252:514-6.
64. Honda GD, Bernstein L, Ross LK, Greenland S, Gerkins V, Henderson B. Vasectomy, cigarette smoking and age at first sexual intercourse as risk factors for prostate cancer in middle-aged men. *Br J Cancer* 1988;57:326-31.
65. Rotkin I. Studies in the epidemiology of prostate cancer: expanded sampling. *Cancer Treat Rep* 1977;61:173-80.
66. Ross R, Deapen DM, Casagrande JT, Paganini-Hill A, Henderson BE. A cohort study of mortality from cancer of the prostate in Catholic priests. *Br J Cancer* 1981;43:233-5.
67. Armenian HK, Lilienfield AM, Diamond EL, Bross ID. Relation between benign prostatic hyperplasia and cancer of the prostate. A prospective and retrospective study. *Lancet* 1974;2:115-7.
68. Nomura A, Kolonel LN. Prostate cancer: a current perspective. *Am J Epidemiol* 1991;13:200-27.
69. McNeal JE. Zonal anatomy of the prostate. *Prostate* 1981;1:35-49.
70. Kjellstrom T, Friberg L, Rahnster B. Mortality and cancer morbidity among cadmium exposed workers. *Lancet* 1983;1:1425-7.
71. Thum M, Schnorr T, Smith AB, et al. Mortality among a cohort of U.S. cadmium production workers: an update. *J Natl Cancer Inst* 1985;74:325-33.
72. Sorahan T, Waterhouse JA. Cancer of prostate among nickel–cadmium battery workers [letter]. *Lancet* 1985;1:459.
73. Armstrong BG, Kazantzis G. The mortality of cadmium workers. *Lancet* 1983;1:1425-7.
74. Aronson KJ, Siemiatycki J, Dewar R, Gérin M. Occupational risk factors for prostate cancer: results from a case–control study in Montréal, Québec, Canada. *Am J Epidemiol* 1996;143:363-73.
75. Gallagher RP, Threlfall WJ, Jeffries E, Band PR, Spinelli J, Coldman AJ. Cancer and aplastic anemia in British Columbia farmers. *J Natl Cancer Inst* 1984;72:1311-5.
76. Burmeister L, Everett G, Van Lier S, Isaacson P. Selected cancer mortality and farm practises in Iowa. *J Occup Med* 1983;118:72-7.
77. Elghany N, Schumacher M, Slattery M, West DW, Lee JS. Occupation, cadmium exposure and prostate cancer. *Epidemiology* 1990;1:107-15.
78. Band PR, Le N, Fang R, Deschamps M, Coldman A, Gallagher RP, et al. Cohort study of Air Canada pilots: mortality, incidence and leukemia risk. *Am J Epidemiol* 1996;143:137-43.
79. Gilliland FD, Mandel JS. Mortality among employees of a perfluorooctanoic acid production plant. *J Occup Med* 1993;35:950-4.
80. American Urological Association. Early detection of prostate cancer [policy statement]. Baltimore: The Association. Available: auanet.org/pub_pat/policies/uroservices .html#Early detection of prostate (accessed 1999 Apr 21).

Appendix 1: Studies of dietary fat and prostate cancer

Site of study	Diagnosis period	Type of study	No. of subjects Cases	No. of subjects Controls	Source of fat (intake)	Summary RR (and 95% CI) in highest exposure group
Japan[19]	1966–1975	Cohort	63	–	Meat	0.9 (NS)
New York[20]	1957–1965	Case–control	311	294	Total fat	2.04 (CI not given, $p < 0.05$)
Kyoto, Japan[21]	1981–1984	Case–control	100	100	Total fat	1.33 (NS, $p > 0.05$)
Washington, DC[22]	1982–1984	Case–control	55	55	Total fat	No difference, RR not given
California[23]	1977–1980	Case–control	142	142	Total fat	1.9 (CI not given, $p < 0.05$)
Hawaii[24]	1977–1983	Case–control	452	899	Saturated fat	1.70 (1.0–2.8)
New York[25]	1982–1988	Case–control	371	371	Annual fat	1.26 (0.76–2.07)
Hawaii[26]	1965–1986	Cohort	174	–	Saturated fat	1.00 (0.75–1.60)
California[27]	1976–1982	Cohort	180	–	Beef	1.21 (0.83–1.75)
Minnesota[28]	1966–1986	Cohort	149	–	Meat	0.8 (0.5–1.3)
Utah[29]	1984–1985	Case–control	358	679	Total fat	Aggressive cases 2.9 (1.0–8.4)
US[30]	1986–1990	Cohort	300	–	Total fat Red meat	Advanced cases 1.79 (1.04–3.07) Advanced cases 2.6 (1.21–5.77)
Sweden[31]	1989–1992	Case–control	256	252	Total fat	0.7 (0.4–1.1)
US and Canada[32]	1987–1991	Case–control	1655	1645	Saturated fat	Aggressive cases 2.8 (1.5–5.2)
Ontario[33]	1990–1992	Case–control	207	207	Total fat	0.7 (0.4–1.3)
Serbia[34]	1990–1994	Case–control	101	202	Total fat	1.95 (0.68–5.57)

Note: RR = relative risk, CI = confidence interval, NS = not significant.

Appendix 2: Studies of β-carotene or vitamin A and prostate cancer

Site of study	Diagnosis period	Type of study	No. of subjects Cases	No. of subjects Controls	Source (intake or level)	Summary RR (and 95% CI) in highest exposure group
New York[20]	1957–1965	Case–control	311	294	Vitamin A	Age < 70, 1.64 (CI not given) Age ≥ 70, 1.97 (CI not given)
Washington, DC[22]	1982–1984	Case–control	55	55	Vitamin A	NS, RR not given
California[23]	1977–1980	Case–control	142	142	Vitamin A	Black men 0.8 (NS) White men 0.9 (NS)
					Carotene	Black men 0.6 (NS) White men 1.0 (NS)
Hawaii[24]	1977–1983	Case–control	452	899	Vitamin A	Age < 70, 0.8 (0.5–1.3) Age ≥ 70, 2.0 (1.3–3.1)
					Carotene	Age < 70, 1.0 (0.6–1.6) Age ≥ 70, 1.5 (0.9–2.3)
California[36]	1981–1986	Cohort	93	–	Total vitamin Dietary carotene	1.2* 1.0*
Rotterdam, Netherlands[37]	1982–1985	Case–control	133	130	Serum retinol level Serum carotene level	0.36 ($p = 0.04$) 0.77 (NS)
Kyoto, Japan[21]	1981–1984	Case–control	100	100	Dietary carotene	0.34 ($p < 0.05$)*
US[38]	1971–1988	Cohort	84	–	Prospective serum vitamin A level	0.4*
Minnesota[28]	1966–1986	Cohort	149	–	Vitamin A	Age < 75, 2.8 (1.4–5.8) Age ≥ 75, 0.4 (0.2–0.9)
					Carotene	Age < 75, 1.9 (1.0–3.7) Age ≥ 75, 0.2 (0.1–0.6)
Utah[29]	1984–1985	Case–control	358	679	Vitamin A	Age 45–67, 1.0 (0.6–1.7) Age 68–74, 1.6 (0.9–2.7)
					Carotene	Age 45–67, 0.8 (0.5–1.2) Age 68–74, 1.4 (0.9–2.4)
US and Canada[32]	1987–1991	Case–control	1655	1645	Vitamin A	No association, RR not given
US[39]	1986–1992	Cohort	773	–	Total retinol equivalents Retinol without supplements	1.13 (0.88–1.44) 1.30 (1.03–1.66)
Serbia[34]	1990–1994	Case–control	101	202	Retinol Retinol equivalent	0.69 (0.50–1.24) 1.64 (1.01–2.67)
Chicago[40]	1957–1989	Cohort	132	–	Carotene	1.03 (0.59–1.60)

*Calculated from data provided in paper.

4

Screening

François Meyer, MD, DSc; Yves Fradet, MD

> A health-conscious 62-year-old man with a recent history of angina is in his general practitioner's office for a scheduled follow-up visit. While vacationing in the United States, he heard about a new test for prostate cancer and wonders if he should have one. His search for information at the library and on the World Wide Web has left him perplexed. He stopped smoking recently, feels well and has no urinary symptoms. His wife, who undergoes mammography regularly, is encouraging him to have the test. He is now seeking his physician's advice.

Physicians' opinions differ on the meaning of the word "screening." To clarify our discussion here, we are adopting Morrison's definition,[1] in which the setting and circumstances of testing are irrelevant:

> Screening for disease control can be defined as the examination of asymptomatic people in order to classify them as likely, or unlikely, to have the disease that is the object of screening.

Others distinguish screening from case finding.[2] For them, "screening" applies only when people are invited to participate in mass testing programs or to visit their physician's office for an annual checkup or periodic health examination, whereas "case finding" refers to screening tests administered to patients who are consulting the physician for

> **KEY POINTS**
> - The prostate-specific antigen (PSA) test is easy to administer, reproducible and inexpensive. Its cancer detection capability is superior to that of digital rectal examination (DRE) alone.
> - Although PSA screening is not advocated by medical organizations in Canada, it is routinely used.
> - The estimated sensitivity and specificity of PSA testing combined with DRE for prostate cancer screening are similar to those of the most sensitive screening strategy for breast cancer.

unrelated illnesses or problems. In the context of the Canadian health care system, such a distinction is confusing, because there are very few organized mass screening programs and annual checkups are no longer recommended.[3] Therefore, screening is usually done in the physician's office during a visit for unrelated reasons, and, in most instances, the terms "case finding" and "screening" represent the same reality.

In Canada decisions on screening are generally made in the physician's office. Proposing a test for screening carries a greater ethical responsibility for the physician than requesting the same test for the diagnostic investigation of symptoms. In screening, the physician initiates the process and bears the responsibility that benefit will follow. Clinicians should be prepared to discuss this issue with their patients, to share uncertainties with them, to listen to their concerns and preferences, and to provide individual counselling.

Evaluation of screening tests

Since the early 1990s, when the prostate-specific antigen (PSA) test became available, screening for prostate cancer has received considerable attention from the medical profession and the public. The PSA test is attractive because of its simplicity, objectivity, reproducibility, lack of invasiveness and relatively low cost. Its cancer detection capability is superior to that of the digital rectal examination (DRE),[4] which has commonly been recommended for the early detection of prostate cancer.

In 1994 the US Food and Drug Administration approved the use of the PSA test in conjunction with DRE as an aid in detecting prostate cancer. Although no Canadian medical organization has come out in favour of screening for prostate cancer,[5] such screening is widely advocated in the United States, especially by the American College of Radiology, the American Urological Association and the American Cancer Society. All of these organizations recommend the combined use of PSA and DRE for screening for prostate cancer. Men with a PSA level over 4 ng/mL, a DRE that raises suspicions of prostate cancer (or both) undergo further examination by transrectal ultrasonography (TRUS) and biopsy. This screening strategy has been used in several programs[6,7] and is being evaluated in the prostate, lung, colorectal and ovarian cancer screening trial of the US National Cancer Institute.[8]

To estimate the sensitivity and specificity of the combination of PSA testing and DRE, we obtained data from the American Cancer Society's National Prostate Cancer Detection Project[4] and the European Randomized Study of Screening for Prostate Cancer,[9] in which every participant also undergoes TRUS (Table 1). For comparison, we abstracted similar data for 50- to 59-year-old women, who were chosen at random for screening by both mammography and physical examination in the Canadian National Breast Screening Study[10] (Table 2).

The data in Tables 1 and 2 were used to estimate the validity of the screening tests for prostate and breast cancer (Table 3). Sensitivity is the ratio of the number of people with a positive test result to the total number of people with the disease in the screened population. For prostate cancer, for the data in Table 1, this ratio is 197/226. It is difficult to identify with certainty all cases of cancer present at the time of screening, including those missed by the test. Different methods, based on different assumptions, have been proposed to resolve this problem. For prostate cancer, we considered all cancers found by biopsy in men with abnormal PSA, DRE or TRUS results as cancers present at the time of screening. For breast cancer, we considered all cancers identified in women with a positive test result plus interval cancers

Table 1: Outcome of initial screening for prostate cancer by prostate-specific antigen (PSA) testing and digital rectal examination (DRE) in 7223 men 55–74 years of age[4,9]

Test result	Status of cancer; no. of men		Total
	Present	Absent	
Positive*	197	1169	1366
Negative	29†	5828	5857
Total	226	6997	7223

*A positive test result corresponds to a PSA level of more than 4 ng/mL, a suspicious DRE result or both.
†Men with a false-negative screening test result are those in whom prostate cancer was discovered by biopsy after transurethral ultrasonography yielded abnormal findings.

Table 2: Outcome of initial screening for breast cancer by mammography and physical examination in 19 711 women 50–59 years of age[10]

Test result	Status of cancer; no. of women		Total
	Present	Absent	
Positive*	142	3 230	3 372
Negative	15†	16 324	16 339
Total	157	19 554	19 711

*A positive test result corresponds to a suspicious finding by mammography, physical examination or both.
†Women with a false-negative screening test result are those in whom breast cancer was discovered during the first year of follow-up (interval cancers).

Table 3: Validity measures of screening tests for prostate and breast cancer

Validity measure	Prostate cancer	Breast cancer
Sensitivity, %	87.2	90.4
Specificity, %	83.3	83.5
Positive test results, %	18.9	17.1
Prevalence of cancer, %	3.1	0.8
Predictive value of a positive test result, %	14.4	4.2

> **KEY POINTS**
> - In the absence of solid evidence of the efficacy of screening, patients and their physicians must make decisions on the basis of personal values and preferences such as the patient's fear of cancer, the potential complications of treatment and the effect of those complications on the patient's quality of life.
> - The progression of prostate cancer after radical prostatectomy can be predicted on the basis of tumour grade, clinical stage and pretreatment PSA level, but not on the basis of the patient's age or tumour volume.

diagnosed in the following year as cancers present at the time of screening. The estimated sensitivity of screening for prostate cancer with PSA testing and DRE was 87.2%, whereas that for screening for breast cancer with mammography and physical examination was 90.4%.

The specificity of screening is the ratio of the number of people free of the disease who have a negative test result to the total number of people free of the disease in the screened population (in Table 1, 5828/6997). For the data presented in Tables 1 and 2, specificity was the same for prostate cancer (83.3%) and breast cancer (83.5%).

Thus, the estimated sensitivity and specificity of the combined screening tests for prostate cancer are similar to those of the most sensitive screening strategy for breast cancer. For both cancer sites, these measures are based on healthy asymptomatic subjects responding to an invitation to participate in a screening study.

Evaluation of screening programs

The predictive value of a positive test result is an important measure that is usually considered in the evaluation of a screening program. It is defined as the ratio of the number of people with a positive test result who have the disease to the total number of people with a positive test result (in Table 1, 197/1366). The predictive value of a positive test result is influenced by the sensitivity and the specificity of the screening test and by the prevalence of the disease at the detectable preclinical phase in the screened population. The prevalence of cancer at the detectable preclinical phase is much higher for prostate cancer than for breast cancer (3.1% v. 0.8%), as is the predictive value of a positive test result (14.4% v. 4.2%). The proportion of test results that were positive (18.9%), the prevalence of cancer (3.1%) and the predictive value of a positive test result for prostate cancer (14.4%) in these studies were slightly lower than those observed in 3 other screening programs using PSA and DRE:[11] 18% to 26%, 3.5% to 4.0% and 15% to 21% respectively. Therefore, on the basis of the validity measures of the screening tests and the characteristics of the screening programs, screening for prostate cancer appears even more promising than screening for breast cancer.

Is screening beneficial?

Comparison of the survival rate for cases detected by screening with that for clinically diagnosed cases is flawed because of several biases: selection, overdiagnosis, lead time and length bias. The randomized controlled trial is the only study design that overcomes these biases and provides a valid assessment of the efficacy of screening in reducing disease-specific mortality rates. Over the past 30 years, randomized controlled trials of breast cancer screening with mammography and clinical breast examination have provided overwhelming evidence that screening in women 50–69 years of age reduces breast cancer mortality rates. In contrast, there are no published data on the efficacy of screening for prostate cancer.

Two major randomized trials are underway, the prostate, lung, colorectal and ovarian cancer screening trial[8] and the European Randomized Study of Screening for Prostate Cancer.[9] The first is an efficacy trial in which 37 000 men aged 60–74 years are being screened annually for 4 years for prostate, lung and colorectal cancer. An equal number of men are being followed with routine medical care as controls. Both PSA testing and DRE are being used in the screening for prostate cancer. A 10-year follow-up of all trial participants will be carried out to determine the effect of screening on prostate cancer mortality rate. Recruitment for the trial started in 1993. The European Randomized Study of Screening for Prostate Cancer is another efficacy trial, started in 1994, in which PSA, DRE and TRUS are being used for screening. The age eligibility criteria and the frequency of rescreening vary from centre to centre. A total of 135 000 men will be recruited into the trial and followed for 10 years. An international collaboration has been established to pool the data from all prostate cancer screening trials to increase statistical power and provide results as early as possible.[12]

Waiting for trial results

These trials in the United States and Europe will not provide a first estimate of the efficacy of screening for prostate cancer before the year 2006. Furthermore, the expected statistical power of the trials will be reduced by poor compliance in the screening arm, contamination in the control arm and an overall downward trend in prostate cancer mortality rates.[13] Thus, there is concern that the question of whether screening for prostate cancer reduces death from that disease will not be answered until much later — if ever.

While waiting for the results of trials in other countries, all Canadian organizations that have adopted a position on the prostate cancer screening issue recommend that patients who request screening be given objective information about the potential benefits and adverse effects of early detection and treatment of prostate cancer so that they can make an informed decision. Some men may experience adverse effects from screening (e.g., those with a false-positive test, those with a false-negative test and those in whom earlier detection of cancer does not result in postponement of death), whereas other men might benefit from screening (only those whose death is postponed because of screening and treatment). It is assumed that men considering screening for prostate cancer and their physicians have enough information to weigh the expected good and harm. The main difficulty with this position is the current absence of any data on the only worthwhile benefit from screening: the reduction of deaths from prostate cancer. Therefore, it is likely that a man's decision to undergo screening for prostate cancer will rest on beliefs rather than objective information.

In evaluating screening programs, it is common practice to consider the 10 criteria proposed by the World Health Organization (Table 4).[14] Screening for prostate cancer clearly satisfies 5 of these criteria, but the status of the other 5 remains uncertain. Furthermore, none of these criteria directly addresses the fundamental question of whether screening reduces the mortality rate of the disease in the screened population.

Prostate cancer is unquestionably an important public health problem. It has a long, detectable, preclinical phase, especially when PSA testing is used for screening. In the Physicians' Health Study, a prospective study of 22 000 physicians in the United States, PSA was measured in stored blood samples.[15] PSA testing up to 4 years before diagnosis would have detected the disease in 73% of the cases of prostate cancer that occurred in this group. The average lead time was 5.5 years, which suggests that the average detectable preclinical phase of prostate cancer exceeds 10 years.[1] This would make screening for prostate cancer very attractive, because the testing would not have to be repeated every year, but possibly only every 5 years or more.

We have a good understanding of the natural history of prostate cancer. The fear that PSA screening would detect a great number of latent cancers

Table 4: Assessment of screening for prostate cancer on the basis of World Health Organization criteria[14]

Criterion	For prostate cancer
Is the disease an important health problem?	Yes
Is there an accepted (effective) treatment for patients with the disease?	Probably
Are there facilities for diagnosis and treatment?	Yes
Is there a detectable preclinical phase of the disease?	Yes
Is there a suitable screening test?	Yes
Is the screening test acceptable to the population?	Yes
Is the natural history of the disease adequately understood?	Partially
Is there a generally accepted strategy to determine which patients should be treated?	To some degree
Are the costs generated by the screening program acceptable?	Possibly
Is there a program for continuous screening?	Premature

that would never have progressed to clinically significant tumours[5,16] now appears unfounded; most prostate cancers detected by PSA screening have been considered clinically significant.[15,17] Furthermore, the detection rates for latent cancer appear to be similar for prostate and breast cancer screening.[18] The concern that there is no way of predicting which screening-detected cancer would have progressed to cause significant morbidity and death[5,16] now appears somewhat overstated. Tumour grade, clinical stage and pretreatment PSA level have been shown to predict independently the progression of prostate cancer after radical prostatectomy,[19] whereas age and tumour volume have not.[11]

There is now some evidence that radical prostatectomy is an effective treatment for the disease. A prospective study of about 60 000 patients treated for prostate cancer in the United States between 1983 and 1992 showed that men referred for radical prostatectomy had a better 10-year survival rate than those for whom the initial treatment decision was radiotherapy or expectant management, particularly for patients with poorly differentiated tumours.[20] The frequency and severity of the adverse side effects of radical treatments are well known. However, many men would gladly accept the risk of iatrogenic impotence and incontinence if radical treatment spares them the pain of metastatic prostate cancer and postpones their death.

This is why it is so important to clearly determine the efficacy of screening in reducing prostate cancer mortality rates. For the first time in record-keeping history, mortality rates from prostate cancer are decreasing in the United States,[21] and a similar trend could be occurring in Canada.[22] This reduction is probably a consequence of better patient management and improved treatment not only for localized tumours but also for advanced prostate cancer. Because prostate cancer mortality rates declined relatively early after the initiation of widespread screening with PSA testing, it is unlikely that screening has contributed to the observed decline.

In the case described at the beginning of this article, the physician can explain that screening for PSA is a good test that detects clinically significant prostate cancers. He can reassure the patient that surgery can improve the survival of men with localized tumours. At the same time, the physician will have to warn the patient that if screening yields a positive result, he may have to face cancer, its treatments and their consequences sooner. Thus the decision as to whether to undergo screening for prostate cancer depends on the patient's personal values and preferences — his fear of cancer, the potential complications of treatment and the impact of those complications on quality of life — in the current absence of proof that screening will delay or prevent death from prostate cancer.

References

1. Morrison AS. *Screening in chronic disease.* New York: Oxford University Press; 1985. p. 3.

2. Sackett DL, Haynes RB, Guyatt GH, Tugwell P. *Clinical epidemiology: a basic science for clinical medicine.* 2nd ed. Boston: Little, Brown; 1991. p. 153.
3. Introduction. In: Canadian Task Force on the Periodic Health Examination. *The Canadian guide to clinical preventive health care.* Ottawa: Health Canada; 1994. p. x.
4. Mettlin C, Murphy GP, Ray P, Shanberg A, Toi A, Chesley A, et al. American Cancer Society: National Prostate Cancer Detection Project. *Cancer* 1993;71:891-8.
5. Feightner JW. Screening for prostate cancer. In: Canadian Task Force on the Periodic Health Examination. *The Canadian guide to clinical preventive health care.* Ottawa: Health Canada; 1994. p. 812-23.
6. Catalona WJ, Smith DS, Ratliff TL, Basler JW. Detection of organ-confined prostate cancer is increased through prostate-specific antigen-based screening. *JAMA* 1993;270:948-54.
7. Labrie F, Dupont A, Suburu R, Cusan L, Gomez JL, Kouytsilieris M, et al. Optimized strategy for detection of early stage, curable prostate cancer: role of prescreening with prostate-specific antigen. *Clin Invest Med* 1994;16:426-41.
8. Gohagan JK, Prorok PC, Kramer BS, Hayes RB, Cornett JE. The prostate, lung, colorectal, and ovarian cancer screening trial of the National Cancer Institute. *Cancer* 1995;75:1869-73.
9. Schröder FH. The European screening study for prostate cancer. *Can J Oncol* 1994; 4(Suppl):102-9.
10. Miller AB, Baines CJ, To T, Wall C. Canadian National Breast Screening Study: 2. Breast cancer detection and death rates among women aged 50 to 59 years. *CMAJ* 1992;147:1477-88.
11. Coley MC, Barry MJ, Fleming C, Mulley AG. Early detection of prostate cancer. Part I: Prior probability and effectiveness of tests. *Ann Intern Med* 1997;126:394-406.
12. Auvinen A, Rietbergen JBW, Denis LJ, Schröder FH, Prorok PC. Prospective evaluation plan for randomized trials of prostate cancer screening. *J Med Screening* 1996;3:97-104.
13. National Cancer Institute. Cancer death rate declined for the first time ever in the 1990s [press release]. 1996 Nov 14. Available: rex.nci.nih.gov/massmedia/pressreleases/cancerdecline.htm (accessed 22 April 1999).
14. Wilson JMG, Jungner G. *Principles and practice of screening for disease.* Geneva: World Health Organization; 1969. Public Health Paper 34.
15. Gann PH, Hennekens CH, Stampfer MJ. A prospective evaluation of plasma prostate-specific antigen for detection of prostatic cancer. *JAMA* 1995;273:289-94.
16. Green CJ, Hadom D, Bassett K, Kazanjian A. *Prostate specific antigen in the early detection of prostate cancer.* Vancouver: British Columbia Office of Health Technology Assessment; 1993.
17. Epstein JI, Walsh PC, Carmichael M, Brendler CB. Pathological and clinical findings to predict tumor extent of nonpalpable (stage T1c) prostate cancer. *JAMA* 1994;271:368-74.
18. Benoit RM, Naslund MJ. Detection of latent prostate cancer from routine screening: comparison with breast cancer screening. *Urology* 1995;46:533-7.
19. Zagars GK, Pollack A, von Eschenbach AC. Prognostic factors for clinically localized prostate carcinoma. *Cancer* 1997;79:1370-80.
20. Lu-Yao GL, Yao SL. Population-based study of long-term survival in patients with clinically localised prostate cancer. *Lancet* 1997;349:906-10.
21. Wingo PA, Ries LAG, Rosenberg HM, Miller DS, Edwards BK. Cancer incidence and mortality, 1973–1995: a report card for the U.S. *Cancer* 1998;82:1197-207.
22. Meyer F, Moore L, Bairati I, Fradet Y. Quebec prostate mortality dropped in 1996. *Cancer Prev Control* 1998;2:163-6.

5

Diagnostic tools for early detection

Pierre I. Karakiewicz, MD; Armen G. Aprikian, MD

A 65-year-old otherwise healthy man is referred for a urologic assessment by his family physician. He has a 1-year history of mildly decreased urinary stream and occasional urgency. The results of a digital rectal examination performed by the referring physician are reported as "unremarkable." Urinalysis demonstrates no abnormal findings. The serum prostate-specific antigen level is 4.6 ng/mL, but 1 year ago it was only 3.8 ng/mL. Transrectal ultrasonography reveals a prostate of normal ultrasonic appearance. No hypoechoic lesion is seen in the peripheral zone. The volume is estimated at 38 cm^3. According to the ultrasound report, biopsy was not performed because of the normal appearance of the prostate.

Diagnosis of prostate cancer at an early stage, when the lesion is localized and curable, followed by effective, definitive therapy, is essential to reduce the number of deaths from this disease.[1] Definitive studies to prove that early detection and treatment reduce the mortality rate have been initiated;[2,3] however, only indirect evidence suggesting the effectiveness of treatment is available.[4] Those in favour of screening for prostate cancer, irrespective of symptoms, recommend an annual serum prostate-specific antigen (PSA) test and digital rectal examination (DRE) for men between the ages of 50 and 70 years.[5] Because of the natural history of the disease, detection is not recommended for men with a life expectancy less than 10 years. For men at high risk for prostate cancer, such as black North Americans and those

KEY POINTS
- Early detection of prostate cancer is of utmost importance, given that localized disease represents the only curable stage. Men with serum levels of prostate-specific antigen (PSA) between 4 and 10 ng/mL constitute the prime target population for effective early detection.
- Although digital rectal examination is the least expensive and most widely used method for detecting prostate cancer, it depends on the skill and subjective assessment of the physician.
- PSA screening should be limited to men at risk of harbouring clinically significant prostate cancer, i.e., men aged 50–70 years (40–70 years in black men and those with a family history of prostate cancer). In selected cases, PSA testing may be performed in men older than 70 years of age if they have longer-than-average life expectancy.

with a family history of prostatic carcinoma, the age range during which testing is recommended is extended to 40 to 70 years.[6]

Our goal here is to take a critical look at the available diagnostic tools that allow detection of prostate cancer in its localized, curable form. We will demonstrate and discuss the following points:
- PSA and DRE represent the most widely used initial evaluation methods.
- Transrectal ultrasonography (TRUS) of the prostate allows visualization of the gland and is required for adequate needle positioning if biopsy is performed.
- TRUS-guided core biopsy of the prostate has become the most widely used and the most definitive means of tissue diagnosis.
- Although classified as prostate cancer staging tools, computed tomography (CT)[7] and magnetic resonance imaging (MRI)[8] of the prostate have not compared favourably with TRUS for early diagnosis.

Digital rectal examination

DRE is the simplest, least expensive and most widely used method for detecting prostate cancer. However, it is highly subjective.[9] Because of this and the differing levels of skill of examiners, many men may be excluded from further assessment because of DRE findings that mimic benign, age-related changes. DRE may also fail to detect cancers of the anterior prostate, which are inaccessible to palpation but contribute to 25% of prostatic malignancy.[10] In addition, 50% of clinically palpable prostatic cancers will either not be amenable to complete surgical excision or will demonstrate local extension before such an attempt.[11] Thus, although DRE constitutes an important diagnostic tool, it may fail to identify a substantial proportion of clinically significant cancers at an organ-confined, curable stage. Further investigation is recommended for any man with DRE findings that raise suspicions of cancer.

Serum prostate-specific antigen test

Testing for serum PSA, a normal serine protease produced by the prostate epithelium, has replaced the relatively insensitive prostatic acid phosphatase test. The function of PSA is to lyse proteins derived from the seminal vesicle; it thus causes semen liquefaction. Under normal conditions, only a small fraction of the PSA produced leaks back from the prostatic acini and ducts to become detectable in the serum.[11]

Conditions that disrupt the junctions thought to prevent leakage of PSA into the serum[12] include prostate cancer, benign prostatic hyperplasia and prostatitis. Urinary retention, prolonged urethral catheterization, recent cystoscopy or prostatic biopsy may also increase circulating PSA levels temporarily.[13] DRE and ejaculation have not been associated with clinically significant elevation of PSA. Drugs that affect the conversion of testosterone to dihydrotestosterone, such as finasteride, reduce circulating serum PSA by about 50%.[14]

When DRE does not raise a suspicion of cancer, serum PSA testing becomes pivotal in establishing the need for TRUS and TRUS-guided core biopsy (Table 1). Serum PSA levels can be determined with either a polyclonal or a monoclonal assay. (The antibodies used in the polyclonal assay react with several epitopes on the PSA molecule, whereas a monoclonal assay is directed against one specific epitope.) At present, monoclonal PSA assays are most common. The normal range of PSA determined by the polyclonal assay is 0 to 2.5 ng/mL,[15] whereas the normal range determined by a monoclonal assay is 0 to 4.0 ng/mL. The polyclonal assay is currently performed in only a few laboratories, and its use will likely be further restricted with the advent of newer forms of PSA testing that rely on monoclonal measurement of the concentration of free and complexed serum PSA. Consequently, only the monoclonal immunoassay will be further discussed here.

Although serum PSA is currently the best clinically available tumour marker, it is not specific to prostate cancer.[16] For example, elevation of PSA

Table 1: Recommended diagnostic tests for various digital rectal examination (DRE) findings and levels of serum prostate-specific antigen (PSA)

Test; findings		
DRE	Serum PSA level, ng/mL	Recommended diagnostic test
Normal	≤ 4.0	Observation, including annual DRE and PSA test
Normal	> 4.0	TRUS and TRUS-guided systematically distributed sector biopsy, as well as biopsy of ultrasonically suspicious areas
Suspicious	Any level	TRUS and TRUS-guided biopsy, including biopsy of palpably or ultrasonically abnormal areas, as well as systematically distributed sector biopsy

Note: TRUS = transrectal ultrasonography.

occurs in 20% to 50% of men with benign prostatic hyperplasia. The test's limitations in sensitivity also account for the discovery of cancer on TRUS-guided core biopsy in as many as 10% of men with PSA values between 0 and 4.0 ng/mL. However, as many as 2 out of 3 men with PSA values greater than 10 ng/mL will be found to have cancer regardless of DRE findings.[17] The current recommendation is that men with serum PSA levels above 4 ng/mL be referred for further evaluation by a urologist. In general, the next diagnostic test consists of TRUS-guided needle biopsy of the prostate.

The limitations in sensitivity and specificity of serum PSA testing have led to attempts to improve its clinical usefulness. New concepts include PSA density, age-specific PSA ranges and PSA velocity, as well as measurements of the proportions of free and bound PSA (Table 2).

PSA density

PSA density, the initial refinement of the PSA test, is an index calculated by dividing total serum PSA by the volume of the prostate, measured ultrasonically by TRUS. In the absence of cancer, prostatic volume is

Table 2: Summary of currently available types of PSA tests			
Diagnostic test	Sensitivity, %	Specificity, %	Comments
Traditional PSA	72–90	59–90	Based on cut-off level of 4.0 ng/mL. Remains standard with which modified forms of PSA testing are compared, although percentage of free PSA appears to offer significant advantages
PSA density	91*	63*	Because of the variability in its performance, which depends on prostate size, this method has fallen out of favour
PSA velocity	61–67†	71–99†	Low sensitivity compared with traditional PSA testing and PSA density. Specificity is superior and increases with increasing follow-up time. However, PSA velocity is often impractical because of long follow-up time required (at least 1.5 to 2 years to maintain adequate specificity)
Age-specific PSA ranges	Improvement of 11% over traditional PSA test	Reduction of 9% compared with traditional PSA test	Because of lower cut-off for men aged 40–49 years, this method offers sensitivity superior to that of traditional PSA testing. Although its overall specificity is lower than that of traditional PSA testing, age-specific PSA also offers better specificity in men aged 70–79 years
% free PSA	90% or greater	Up to 80%	Still an investigational tool. Can increase the specificity of traditional PSA testing, especially in the diagnostic "grey zone," between 4 and 10 ng/mL. No consensus on cut-off value

*Based on the suggested cut-off value of 0.15 ng/mL PSA per cubic centimetre of prostate tissue.
†Based on a cut-off value of 0.75 ng/mL annually.

directly proportional to circulating serum PSA.[18] Benign prostatic hyperplasia is associated with, on average, only 0.26 ng/mL PSA per gram of tissue, whereas cancer results in a density 10-fold higher.[19] Any PSA value greater than that predicted by gland volume should raise a suspicion of prostate cancer.

The optimal cut-off value for PSA density is a trade-off between sensitivity and biopsy rate. A low cut-off value yields high sensitivity and better detection but corresponds to a higher rate of potentially unnecessary biopsies. The opposite is true with a higher cut-off value. Because 2 out of 3 men with a PSA level between 4 and 10 ng/mL are found by prostate biopsy not to have cancer, PSA density is used to identify those who should not undergo unnecessary biopsy. Because a PSA density of less than 0.15 ng/mL per cubic centimetre of prostatic tissue is associated with a low likelihood of cancer, this the most widely used cut-off point.[20]

> **KEY POINTS**
> - The level of PSA in blood serum is currently the best test for prostate cancer, but limitations in its sensitivity and specificity have led to attempts to improve its clinical usefulness.
> - The PSA density test factors in prostate volume to avoid unnecessary biopsy in men whose prostate is enlarged.
> - Age-specific PSA ranges are based on the assumption that older men have larger prostates and may therefore have higher serum PSA levels not associated with carcinoma.
> - A further refinement of the PSA test — PSA velocity testing — measures the rate of change of serum PSA levels over time.
> - The measurement of free and bound forms of PSA in the serum distinguishes between men with prostate cancer and those with benign prostatic hyperplasia and is the most promising method of increasing the specificity of PSA testing.
> - PSA testing and each of its modifications still necessitate a trade-off between specificity and sensitivity.

The suggested benefit of PSA density derives from the fact that a significant number of men are spared biopsy even though they have PSA levels above 4.0 ng/mL. Although this was initially reported not to result in lack of detection of clinically significant cancers,[20] more recent analyses have demonstrated that the diagnostic accuracy of PSA density is limited because of the inherent limitations of TRUS in determining prostate volume.[21,22] In addition, inadequate sampling in men with prostates larger than 50 to 60 cm^3 may have led to false-negative biopsy results, which may have further undermined the validity of initial PSA density results.[17,23,24] On the basis of these findings, the use of PSA density in clinical practice has declined substantially. Finally, given the minimal morbidity associated with biopsy, the excellent level of patient tolerance associated with this procedure and the requirement to perform TRUS gland volumetry in order to calculate PSA density, performing an ultrasonic assessment without concomitant biopsy is of questionable benefit.

Age-specific PSA ranges

Age-specific PSA ranges, which rely on age instead of TRUS volumetry, are based on the assumption that older men have larger prostates and, therefore, may have higher serum PSA levels not associated with carcinoma. More specifically, the introduction of age-specific PSA ranges was aimed at increasing the sensitivity of PSA testing in younger men and increasing the specificity of such testing in older men.[25] The reference ranges are given in Table 3.

The adoption of these age-specific maximum PSA values has increased the number of biopsies performed in younger men and decreased the number performed in older men. The rationale was to detect more early cancers in the men who could benefit most from definitive therapy, while limiting detection of cancers of questionable clinical significance in men with shorter life expectancy. An additional advantage of age-specific PSA over PSA density is the fact that ultrasonic gland measurement and the associated cost can be avoided. At present, because of the limited data regarding age-specific PSA and the lack of precise guidelines for its clinical use, its role in the early detection of prostate cancer remains unclear.

Table 3: Reference ranges for age-specific PSA levels

Age range, yr	Upper limit of PSA, ng/mL
40–49	2.5
50–59	3.5
60–69	4.5
70–79	6.5

PSA velocity

A further refinement of the single PSA measurement is serial measurements and trend analysis.[26] The term "PSA velocity" refers to the rate of change of serum PSA level over time. Early investigators of this concept demonstrated significant differences in PSA velocity between men with benign prostatic hyperplasia and those with prostate cancer. These differences were detectable as early as 9 years before prostate cancer was diagnosed. Others have confirmed the benefit of PSA velocity over a single PSA measurement.[27] However, at least 3 consecutive measurements are required for reliable calculation of PSA velocity. The optimal interval between these measurements has not yet been determined, but 6 months is currently recommended. Therefore, a follow-up of at least 18 months is necessary to achieve the maximum benefit of PSA velocity in prostate cancer detection.

Problems with PSA velocity include important physiologic and intra-individual variability, reportedly as high as 23.5%.[28] Therefore, if 2 samples are obtained from the same person 2 to 3 weeks apart, the serum PSA level may be 3.5 ng/mL for the first test and 4.3 ng/mL for the subsequent analysis, without any change in the condition of the prostate itself. Similarly, methodological variation in PSA tests may range from 10% to 45%.[29] Thus, if the same serum sample is subjected to analysis by 2 different assays, the PSA level may be 4.0 ng/mL with one assay and between 4.4 and 5.8 ng/mL with the other. These variations may preclude effective use of PSA velocity in large-scale screening.

A potential benefit can be derived from PSA velocity in men with serum PSA values below 4 ng/mL who harbour prostate cancer. In men with normal PSA values, an annual increase in excess of 20%[30] or PSA velocity exceeding 0.75 ng/mL annually[31] is suggestive of prostate cancer and indicates the need for urological evaluation. Determining PSA velocity in men with traditional serum PSA values above the normal upper limit of 4 ng/mL is of little additional benefit, given that a urological assessment is warranted regardless of the rate of increase in PSA level.

Percentage of free PSA

In further efforts to enhance the sensitivity and specificity of PSA testing, the measurement of free and bound forms of PSA in the serum has been proposed. In the serum, PSA complexes predominantly with the α_1 subunit of antichymotrypsin and the α_2 subunit of macroglobulin. Most commercially available complexed-PSA assays determine the concentration of the PSA–antichymotrypsin complex. Nearly all of the remaining circulating PSA is in its free form. The proportion of free PSA is known to be lower in those with prostate cancer than in those with benign prostatic hyperplasia; thus, the likelihood of prostate cancer increases with decreasing free PSA. In contrast, the proportion of free PSA increases with advancing age and increasing prostate volume.

Recent studies have identified the proportion of free PSA as an independent predictor of prostate cancer, superior to both DRE and total PSA level. Likewise, the proportion of free PSA has a superior diagnostic accuracy relative to PSA density.[32] In a recently published large-scale study, determination of the proportion of free PSA would have maintained a specificity of 90% and would have eliminated the need for biopsy in 31.3% of men with benign DRE findings and serum PSA levels between 4 and 10 ng/mL.[33] At present, only free PSA offers high specificity and adequate sensitivity. Consequently, it is the most clinically valuable and most promising modification of the PSA test.

Several recommendations for cut-off levels have emerged. As with all other forms of PSA tests, there is a trade-off between sensitivity and specificity. A cut-off of 23.4% free PSA eliminated 31% of biopsies while maintaining 90% sensitivity.[34] In men with serum PSA values between 2.6 and 4.0 ng/mL, a cut-off point of 27% eliminated 18% of biopsies with a sensitivity greater than 90%. Therefore, proportion of free PSA appears capable of enhancing the sensitivity and specificity of traditional PSA testing, even in men with normal serum PSA levels.[34]

Diagnostic limitations of PSA testing and its enhanced forms

Although results obtained by measuring serum PSA levels are superior in terms of prostate cancer detection to those obtained with any other clinically available tumour marker, the traditional total PSA value and each of its enhanced forms share several limitations. The principal concern is that although diagnostic accuracy has improved with each of the modifications to total serum PSA measurement, none of the forms is specific for prostate cancer. Each requires a trade-off in specificity for increased sensitivity and vice versa. This trade-off appears to be most advantageous with proportion of free PSA. Currently, proportion of free PSA appears to be the best detection tool for men with serum PSA levels below 10 ng/mL and is rapidly approaching routine clinical practice. However, definitive large-scale studies aimed at defining the optimal cut-off value are continuing.[33] Thus, this test remains an investigational tool.

Transrectal ultrasonography

TRUS plays an invaluable role in directing and positioning biopsy needles; however, its direct contribution to detection of prostate cancer is limited. Cancerous lesions are associated with decreased echogenicity if situated within the periphery of the prostate or the posterior aspect of the gland closest to the rectal wall. Malignant lesions can be associated with mixed echogenicity, as well as hypoechoic appearance, if situated within the anterior prostate.[10] Recently, colour-flow Doppler imaging has been introduced in an attempt to detect increased vascularity associated with prostate cancer. Although this method is not specific, it allowed the detection of approximately 7% more cancers than were detected by DRE and TRUS.[35] It has been suggested that the detection of vascular cancers in particular is important as they may be more likely to spread.[36]

Biopsy of suspicious lesions anywhere in the prostate is mandatory, and positive biopsy results in as many as 30% of cases have been reported.[16,17] However, because of the heterogeneity of ultrasonically visible prostatic findings, their interpretation is highly subjective. Consequently, the sensitivity and specificity of TRUS alone in prostate cancer detection is unacceptably low. Therefore, the importance of adequate histologic sampling of the prostate by obtaining multiple core biopsy specimens of both suspicious and visually normal tissue cannot be overemphasized. In the presence of elevated PSA levels, prostatic biopsy is recommended, even if DRE and TRUS findings indicate benignity, because nonpalpable, nonvisible prostate cancer may be found in 40% of such cases.[17]

CT is not useful for early detection of prostate cancer. MRI is about as accurate in detecting early cancer as TRUS but cannot be used to direct biopsy. Its current inaccessibility for timely clinical applications and its high cost preclude its use for early detection. Both CT and MRI can be helpful in staging cancer, because they can indicate periprostatic tumour spread, lymph node abnormality and bone involvement, but their sensitivity for revealing tumour extension has limitations.

> **KEY POINTS**
> - Transrectal ultrasonography of the prostate allows visualization of the gland and is required for adequate needle positioning if biopsy is performed.
> - Transrectal ultrasound-guided core biopsy of the prostate has become the most widely used and the best means of determining the grade, volume and localization of a tumour, as well as its distribution within the prostate.

Prostatic biopsy

Prostatic biopsy represents the cornerstone of prostate cancer diagnosis.[17] It provides valuable information about grade, volume and localization, as well as the distribution of tumour within the prostate.[37] Digitally guided transrectal and transperineal biopsy, although still used occasionally, are associated with dismally low positive biopsy rates compared with TRUS-guided core biopsy.[38] TRUS-guided core biopsy of 6 cores of tissue in addition to cores directed toward palpable or ultrasonically visible abnormalities is the current standard for prostate biopsy. Although associated with some discomfort, TRUS-guided biopsy is performed without anesthesia or sedation and is a well-tolerated procedure with minimal morbidity.[39] Quinolone antibiotic prophylaxis — consisting of 1 dose before biopsy and 4 doses afterward — is usually administered. A study assessing biopsy-related complications reported temperature elevation above 38°C, consistent with infection, in 1.4% of patients who underwent peripheral zone biopsies.[39] The most commonly reported complications consist of traces of blood in the urine, semen or feces. Although reported by most patients, these complications are limited and subside within 2–3 weeks after the procedure. Pain at the time of biopsy is universally reported. However, only in exceptional cases is analgesia or sedation required. As many as 50% of men report significant pain after biopsy, but this usually subsides within 4 days.

Recent reports suggest the need for additional systematic biopsy of glands that seem normal (by both palpation and visualization), which results in denser sampling.[17,23,24,40,41] These reports are based on the observation of suboptimal sampling with sextant biopsy. Lack of detection of clinically significant cancers may occur predominantly in men with prostates in excess of 50 or 60 cm³. An algorithm incorporating prostate size has been advocated to maintain a steady positive biopsy rate throughout the wide range of gland sizes. It has been suggested that as many as one core for each 5 cm³ of prostate tissue may be required for effective detection of clinically localized disease.[42,43] In a rationale similar to that for age-specific PSA levels, patient age may be used to determine the appropriate sampling density.[40] Although sextant biopsy with additional biopsy of palpable or ultrasonically visible lesions is still the most widely used approach, several centres employ a denser biopsy template.[24]

Table 4: Recommended number of cores for prostate biopsy according to prostate size[43]

Prostate size, cm³	No. of cores
≤ 30	6
30.1–40	8
40.1–50	10
50.1–60	12
60.1–70	14
70.1–80	16
> 80	18

In men with normal biopsy results despite elevated serum PSA, we suggest follow-up with serial PSA measurements. Although such repeat PSA measurements are usually obtained at 3- to 6-month intervals, there is no consensus regarding the optimal interval. Should the serial PSA measurements demonstrate rising PSA, repeat biopsy is indicated. Repeat biopsy is also recommended if high-grade prostatic intra-epithelial neoplasia is found in the initial biopsy specimen. The repeat procedure should be performed within 3 months of the initial biopsy. We suggest a denser pattern of sampling, in which the number of cores is determined according to the gland volume (Table 4).[43]

Conclusion

Localized prostate cancer represents the only curable stage of this disease. Therefore, effective detection implies diagnosis at this stage. In view of the elevated rate of locally advanced disease associated with serum PSA levels above 10 ng/mL, men with PSA between 4 and 10 ng/mL constitute the prime target population for effective early detection. However, because of the high prevalence of benign prostatic hyperplasia, which may contribute to intermediate serum PSA elevation (between 4.1 and 10 ng/mL), and normal-appearing DRE results, many physicians delay the required biopsy. Failure to perform biopsy at this time may result in lack of detection of clinically significant disease while it is still at a curable stage.

We have reiterated here the subjectivity of DRE and stress its poor performance when used alone for the early detection of prostate cancer. We have also highlighted the need for PSA testing, especially in the face of normal DRE results. The current recommendations for prostate cancer detection suggest the use of both DRE and serum PSA testing instead of one or the other alone. The usefulness of the traditional PSA cut-off value of 4 ng/mL may be further enhanced: PSA velocity and proportion of free PSA may prove highly beneficial in young, otherwise healthy men. In this patient subgroup, early and effective diagnosis maximizes the long-term benefits of curative therapy. Finally, we have completed this review by restating the central role of prostatic biopsy under TRUS guidance. We have re-emphasized the need for adequate histologic sampling of the prostate once the suspicion of cancer has been entertained. To obtain such valuable diagnostic information as tumour grade, volume, localization and distribution, a minimum of 6 core biopsy samples should be obtained, and several additional biopsy samples are required in patients with large prostate glands, where localization of the malignancy within abundant prostatic tissue is more difficult.

On the basis of the information given in the case presented at the beginning of this article and our discussion of diagnostic methods, the presence of nonpalpable, ultrasonically nonvisible cancer cannot be excluded in this patient. As many as 20% of men fitting this description may harbour prostatic malignancy. Consequently, ultrasonically guided sector biopsies are clearly indicated.

References

1. Catalona WJ. Screening for early detection of prostate cancer [letter]. *Lancet* 1996;347:1629.
2. Gohagan JK, Prorok PC, Kramer BS, Cornett JE. Prostate cancer screening in the prostate, lung, colorectal and ovarian cancer screening trial of the National Cancer Institute. *J Urol* 1994;152:1905-9.
3. Wilt TJ, Brawer MK. The prostate cancer intervention versus observation trial: a randomized trial comparing radical prostatectomy versus expectant management for the treatment of clinically localized prostate cancer. *J Urol* 1994;152:1910-4.
4. Schroeder FH. Screening, early detection and treatment of prostate cancer: a European view. *Urology* 1995;46(3 Suppl A):62-70.
5. Smith DS, Catalona WJ, Herschman JD. Longitudinal screening for prostate cancer with prostate specific antigen. *JAMA* 1996;276:1309-15.
6. Aprikian AG, Bazinet M, Plante M, Meshref A, Trudel C, Aronson S, et al. Family history and the risk of prostatic carcinoma in a high risk group of urological patients. *J Urol* 1995;154:404-6.
7. Platt JF, Bree RL, Schwab RE. The accuracy of CT in the staging of carcinoma of the prostate. *Am J Radiol* 1977;1:281-9.

8. Rifkin MD, Zerhouni EA, Gatsonis CA, Quint LE, Paushter DM, Epstein JI, et al. Comparison of magnetic resonance imaging and ultrasonography in staging early prostate cancer. Results of a multi-institutional cooperative trial. *N Engl J Med* 1990;323:621-6.
9. Smith DS, Catalona WJ. Interexaminer variability of digital rectal examination in detecting prostate cancer. *Urology* 1995;45:70-4.
10. Bazinet M, Karakiewicz PI, Aprikian AG, Trudel C, Aronson S, Nachabé M, et al. Value of systematic transition zone biopsies in the early detection of prostate cancer. *J Urol* 1996;155:605-6.
11. Goldenberg SL, Klotz LH, Srigley J, Jewett MA, Mador D, Fradet Y, et al. Randomized, prospective, controlled study comparing radical prostatectomy alone and neoadjuvant androgen withdrawal in the treatment of localized prostate cancer. Canadian Urologic Oncology Group. *J Urol* 1996;156:873-7.
12. Bostwick DG. Prostate specific antigen: current role in diagnostic pathology of prostate cancer. *Am J Clin Pathol* 1994;102(4 Suppl 1):S31-7.
13. Tchetgen MBN, Oesterling JE. The effect of prostatitis, urinary retention, ejaculation, and ambulation on the serum prostate specific antigen concentration. *Urol Clin North Am* 1997;24:283-91.
14. Guess HA, Gormley GJ, Stoner E, Oesterling JE. The effect of finasteride on prostate specific antigen: review of available data. *J Urol* 1996;155:3-9.
15. Terris MK, Stamey TA. Utilization of polyclonal serum prostate specific antigen levels in screening for prostate cancer: a comparison with corresponding monoclonal values. *Br J Urol* 1994;73:61-4.
16. Partin AW, Oesterling JE. The clinical usefulness of prostate specific antigen: update 1994. *J Urol* 1994;152:1358-68.
17. Karakiewicz PI, Bazinet M, Aprikian AG, Trudel C, Aronson S, Nachabé M, et al. Outcome of sextant biopsy according to gland volume. *Urology* 1997;49:55-9.
18. Benson MC, Whang IS, Pantuck A, Ring K, Kaplan SA, Olsson CA, et al. Prostate specific antigen density: a means of distinguishing benign prostatic hypertrophy and prostate cancer. *J Urol* 1992;147:815-9.
19. Hammerer PG, McNeal JE, Stamey TA. Correlation between serum prostate specific antigen levels and the volume of the individual glandular zones of the human prostate. *J Urol* 1995;153:111-4.
20. Bazinet M, Meshref AW, Trudel C, Aronson S, Peloquin F, Nachabé M, et al. Prospective evaluation of prostate-specific antigen density and systematic biopsies for early detection of prostatic carcinoma. *Urology* 1994;43:44-51.
21. Bazinet M, Karakiewicz PI, Aprikian AG, Trudel C, Aronson S, Nachabé M, et al. Reassessment of non-planimetric transrectal ultrasound prostate volume estimates. *Urology* 1996;47:857-62.
22. Karakiewicz PI, Bazinet M, Aprikian AG, Trudel C, Aronson S, Péloquin F, et al. Analysis of gland volume effect on the performance of PSA density in early detection of non-palpable, isoechoic prostate cancer. *Can J Urol* 1996;3:212-20.
23. Karakiewicz PI, Aprikian AG, Meshref AW, Bazinet M. Computer-assisted comparative analysis of four and six sector biopsies of the prostate. *Urology* 1996;48:747-50.

24. Levine MA, Ittman M, Melamed J, Lepor H. Two consecutive sets of transrectal ultrasound guided sextant biopsies of the prostate for the detection of prostate cancer. *J Urol* 1998;159:471-6.
25. Oesterling JE, Jacobsen SJ, Chute CG, Guess HA, Girman CJ, Panser LA, et al. Serum prostate-specific antigen in a community-based population of healthy men: establishment of age specific reference ranges. *JAMA* 1993;270:860-4.
26. Carter HB, Pearson JD, Metter EJ, Brant LJ, Chan DW, Andres R, et al. Longitudinal evaluation of prostate specific antigen levels in men with and without prostate cancer. *JAMA* 1992;267:2215-7.
27. Catalona WJ, Smith DS, Ratliff TL. Value of measurement of the rate of change of serum PSA levels in prostate cancer screening [abstract 348]. *J Urol* 1993;149:300A.
28. Prestigiacomo AF, Stamey TA. Physiological variation of prostate specific antigen in the 4.0 to 10.0 ng/mL range in male volunteers. *J Urol* 1996;155:1977-80.
29. Nixon RG, Wener MH, Smith KM, Parson RE, Strobel SA, Brawer MK. Biological variation of prostate specific antigen levels in serum: an evaluation of day-to-day physiological fluctuations in a well-defined cohort of 24 patients. *J Urol* 1997;157:2183-90.
30. Brawer MK, Beattie J, Wener MH, Vessella RL, Preston SD, Lange PH. Screening for prostatic carcinoma with prostate specific antigen: results of the second year. *J Urol* 1993;150:106-11.
31. Carter HB, Morrel CH, Pearson JD, Brant LJ, Plato CC, Metter EJ, et al. Estimation of prostatic growth using serial prostate specific antigen measurement in men with and without prostate cancer. *Cancer Res* 1992;52:3323-6.
32. Prestigiacomo AF, Stamey TA. Can free and total prostate specific antigen and prostatic volume distinguish between men with negative and positive systematic ultrasound guided prostate biopsies? *J Urol* 1997;157:189-94.
33. Catalona WJ, Partin AW, Slawin KM, Brawer MK, Patel A, Flanigan RC, et al. A multicenter trial evaluation of free PSA in the differentiation of prostate cancer from benign disease [abstract]. *J Urol* 1997;157:434A.
34. Catalona WJ, Smith DS, Ornstein DK. Prostate cancer detection in men with serum PSA concentrations of 2.6 to 4.0 ng/mL and benign prostate examination. Enhancement of specificity with free PSA measurement. *JAMA* 1997;277:1475-6.
35. Rifkin MD, Sudakoff GS, Alexander AA. Prostate: techniques, results, and the potential applications of colour Doppler. *Radiology* 1993;186:509-13.
36. Alexander AA. To colour Doppler image the prostate or not: that is the question. *Radiology* 1995;195:11-3.
37. Stamey TA. Making the most out of six systematic sextant biopsies. *Urology* 1995;45:2-12.
38. Karakiewicz PI, Bazinet M, Meshref AW, Aprikian AG, Trudel C, Aronson S, et al. Value of repeat ultrasonic prostatic biopsies following negative digitally directed biopsy. *Can J Urol* 1997;4:289-92.
39. Bazinet M, Karakiewicz PI, Aprikian AG, Trudel C, Aronson S, Péloquin F, et al. Complications of ultrasound-guided prostate biopsy peripheral zone only versus peripheral and transition zone biopsy. *Urol Oncol* 1996;2:65-9.
40. Vashi AR, Wojno KJ, Gillespie B, Oesterling JE. Patient age and prostate gland size determine the appropriate number of cores per biopsy [abstract]. *J Urol*

1997;157:1428A.
41. Uzzo RG, Wei JT, Waldbaum RS, Perlmutter AP, Byrne JC, Vaughan ED Jr. The influence of prostate size on cancer detection. *Urology* 1995;46:831-6.
42. Karakiewicz PI, Hanley JA, Bazinet M. Prediction of cancer detection rates with sector biopsy of the prostate: a three dimensional dynamic model [abstract]. *J Urol* 1996;155:259A.
43. Karakiewicz PI, Hanley JA, Bazinet M. Three-dimensional computer-assisted analysis of sector biopsy of the prostate. *Urology* 1998;52:208-12.

6

Surgical treatment of localized disease

S. Larry Goldenberg, MD; Ernest W. Ramsey, MD;
Michael A.S. Jewett, MD

> A 65-year-old man undergoes a routine checkup before retiring. His wife has urged him to have his prostate examined, because she has read about testing for prostate cancer and a friend has just died of this disease. During the rectal examination, the man's physician discovers some firmness in the right lobe of the prostate gland. The patient has had no urinary symptoms and is in excellent general health. Sexual function is normal. There is no family history of prostate cancer; his father died of a stroke at age 86 years. Testing shows that the patient's prostate-specific antigen level is 9.3 ng/mL, and he is referred to a urologist. Transrectal ultrasound-guided needle biopsy reveals adenocarcinoma with a Gleason score of 7 (intermediate grade). At a follow-up meeting with his physician, the patient says, "I have been doing some research, and it appears that I should have treatment. However, what is less clear to me is what form of therapy is best — surgery or radiation treatment. Please tell me what you can about the state of the art with respect to surgery."

The patient described in this case is an appropriate candidate for radical prostatectomy (total removal of the prostate and surrounding tissues). At age 65, in good general health and with a family history of longevity, he has excellent life expectancy. He has clinical stage T2a adenocarcinoma (i.e., it is detectable during digital rectal examination [DRE] but is confined to one lobe of the prostate) with a Gleason score of 7 and a baseline prostate-specific antigen level of 9.3 ng/mL.[1]

Conservative management, such as watchful waiting, is not a good

> **KEY POINTS**
> - Radical prostatectomy is a good option for patients who are otherwise in good health and have a life expectancy of at least 10 years, provided the tumour is confined to the prostate and the level of prostate-specific antigen is less than 20 ng/mL.
> - Radical prostatectomy is a relatively safe procedure; the associated mortality rate is low, and early complications are rare.

option for this patient because of the tumour grade and the elevated PSA. A meta-analysis[2] has indicated that only 26% of men with untreated high-grade prostate cancer survive for 10 years without metastasis. In contrast, if radical prostatectomy is performed at this stage, there is a 33% probability that the disease will be confined to the prostate, a 52% chance of capsular penetration, a 10% likelihood of seminal vesical involvement and only a 4% probability of lymph node involvement.[3] Overall, this patient has a reasonable chance of cure with surgery.

Candidates for radical prostatectomy

In the appropriate patient, radical prostatectomy may be curative, and the procedure is both logically and emotionally appealing. However, it is not for everyone. Suitability for radical prostatectomy is based on several criteria.

- The tumour must appear to be confined to the prostate, that is, stage T1 or T2. If the disease is more advanced, radical prostatectomy is unlikely to be curative, and the risks and side effects of the operation cannot be justified.
- The PSA level should generally be less than 20 ng/mL.
- The patient must be medically fit to withstand anesthesia and major surgery.
- Older age is not an automatic disqualification for surgery, but unless the patient has a life expectancy of at least 10 years, surgery is not likely to improve overall survival. Therefore, prostatectomy is usually performed only in patients under the age of 70 who are otherwise in good health.

When a man discusses the option of prostate removal with his urologist, he needs to be aware of both the benefits and the risks. The potential benefits are clear: the cancer could be completely eradicated and the man cured of the disease. The risks, however, may be considerable. These include the risks of perioperative and postoperative complications, as well as the risks of long-term complications.

Procedures

Once prostate cancer has been confirmed by biopsy, all of the information gathered from the digital rectal examination, the PSA test and nuclear bone scanning is used in staging the tumour. Bone scanning may be omitted if the PSA level is below 10 ng/mL and the Gleason score is less than 7, because the chance of skeletal metastasis in this setting is less than 1%.[4]

For more locally advanced but still clinically confined cancers, some urologists recommend a course of neoadjuvant hormone therapy for a limited time before surgery.[5] Such therapy will cause the prostate, and the cancer within it, to shrink. Studies have confirmed that a 3-month course of treatment significantly improves the odds of achieving negative margins[5] (i.e., "getting it all out"). Current trials are evaluating longer-duration therapy (8 months), and continuing follow-up in all studies is necessary to determine whether this double-barrelled approach will lead to longer survival times.[6] However, it is not routinely recommended at present outside the clinical trial setting.

> **KEY POINTS**
> - Improvements in surgical techniques have reduced the risks of incontinence and erectile dysfunction after prostatectomy.
> - The risk of excessive blood loss during surgery has also declined.
> - Autologous blood donation, which was popular for some time, is expensive and unnecessary for this procedure.
> - Normovolemic hemodilution during surgery — the removal of 2–3 units of blood, dilution of the circulating blood to maintain normal volume and the replacement of the units once blood loss is controlled — is of value.
> - The administration of erythropoietin before surgery may be appropriate for some men with low hematocrit.

Of the 2 techniques used in radical prostatectomy, the most common is radical retropubic prostatectomy. The other option, radical perineal prostatectomy (in which the prostate is approached through an incision in the perineum), has several advantages. These include minimal loss of blood, easier reconstruction of the bladder–urethra connection once the prostate has been removed, and a shorter stay in hospital. The disadvantages are a higher rate of impotence and the inability to assess the state of the lymph nodes near the prostate without a second operation. At present, only a few urologists perform this procedure.

What the patient should know before surgery

At most hospitals, patients attend a preadmission assessment clinic well in advance of their surgery. During this clinic, a variety of admission procedures and laboratory assessments, including a blood crossmatch, are carried out. The patient is then admitted to hospital on the day of surgery.

Because the rectal wall may (rarely) be lacerated during the procedure, the bowel must be cleansed of feces beforehand. Patients are also given antibiotics to minimize the chances of infection. Some surgeons prescribe oral tablets to be started a day or two before surgery; others request intravenous administration of antibiotics to be started just before the operation and to continue for a few days afterward.

What happens during surgery

The first step in the surgical procedure is to examine the regional lymph nodes. If the nodes are obviously abnormal and metastatic tumour is confirmed on quick section, the disease is almost certainly metastatic elsewhere and therefore incurable, so proceeding with the surgery would be inappropriate. However, if the cancer is at an early stage (T1a, T1b or T2a) and is of low grade (Gleason score below 7) and the PSA level is below 10 ng/mL, the probability of metastasis to the lymph nodes is low (less than 5%).[3] In this situation, the surgeon may elect to forego lymph node dissection, thus reducing the operating time and associated intraoperative and postoperative complications. Before the operation begins, it should be clear to both the patient and the surgeon what will be done in any of the situations that might be encountered.

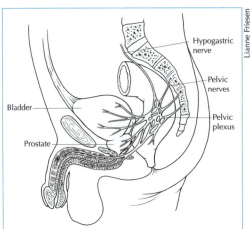

Fig. 1: Side view showing sagittal section of the male pelvis, detailing the normal anatomic features of the prostate region.

Before the 1980s the traditional procedure involved wide resection of the prostate gland and, as a result, 80% to 90% of patients lost their ability to attain an erection. In 1983, the nerve-sparing or anatomic prostatectomy was introduced to minimize the problem of postoperative impotence (Figs. 1–3). In theory, if the nerves are spared on both sides of the prostate, the patient should retain erectile function, and this hypothesis has been borne out particularly among younger patients, in whom some degree of erectile capacity may be preserved in 60% to 70% of cases. However, if the patient is older or has a history of

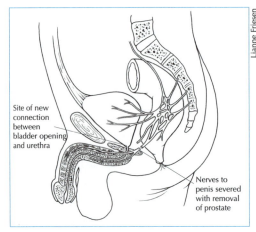

Fig. 2: Side view showing the nerves that are severed during classical radical prostatectomy.

erectile dysfunction, the likelihood of maintaining erectile function after surgery drops dramatically, to approximately 15%.

Nerve-sparing or anatomic prostatectomy should be used only when the cancer does not extend to the edge or the apex of the gland. If there is doubt as to whether the entire cancer can be taken out, a wider margin of tissue must be removed. Ultimately, the preservation of erectile function depends on the patient's age, his current sexual ability, the extent of the cancer, the use of unilateral or bilateral nerve-sparing surgery, and the skill and experience of the surgeon.

During the prostatectomy, special care is also given to the apical dissection. Minimizing the amount of surgical trauma around the external sphincter, the puboprostatic ligaments and the membranous urethra increases the likelihood that the patient will regain full continence at an early stage. It is common for the patient to dribble some urine involuntarily after the catheter is removed, but in most cases this clears up within a few months or even weeks.

Once the prostate has been removed, the bladder neck is anastomosed to the urethra. The catheter must be left in the bladder for 10 to 15 days to allow the newly formed urethral connection to heal. A small drain is inserted to remove any blood or urine that might otherwise collect in the retropubic space in the first days after surgery.

What the patient should expect after surgery

Most patients can tolerate fluids by mouth within a day after surgery, and a regular diet can usually be resumed by the second or third postoperative day — sooner after radical perineal surgery.

Pain after surgery can usually be controlled with narcotic analgesics. Some hospitals offer patient-controlled analgesia, such that the patient can dispense his own medication when he begins to feel pain. A push button activates a pump that delivers a small, preset amount of morphine into the intravenous set, which gives immediate pain relief. In this way, the level of analgesic in the blood is kept relatively constant. Patients using this system actually use less narcotic overall during the postoperative period than those who

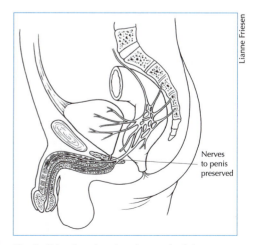

Fig. 3: Side view showing the result of the nerve-sparing procedure.

must rely on other sources. Another option offered by some hospitals is an epidural catheter, which affords excellent analgesia to the pelvis and perineum. Non-narcotic pain medication, which is associated with a lower risk of constipation or paralytic ileus, may be prescribed.

Most patients are ready for discharge on the fourth or fifth day; the catheter, which must remain in place for several more days, is attached to a leg drainage bag.

Early complications

A wide variety of early complications may occur, some specific to this procedure and others that represent the general complications of surgery (Table 1).[7-11]

Blood loss

The prostate is surrounded by an extensive plexus of veins, and blood loss associated with radical prostatectomy has been a major problem. Improvements in surgical techniques related to control of the dorsal venous complex have led to a decline in blood loss. In 1987 Igel and colleagues[8] reported a mean blood loss of 1018 (range 50–7000) mL in a series of 692 patients; in 1992 Leandri and associates[9] reported a mean blood loss of only 300 (range 100–1500) mL in 220 procedures. A review of the 878 radical prostatectomies carried out in Manitoba between 1985 and 1995 indicated that the mean blood loss decreased from 2500–3000 to 1000–1500 mL during that period.[7]

Table 1: Early complications of radical retropubic prostatectomy[7-11]

Complication	Prevalence, %
Pulmonary embolism	0.7–2.7
Deep venous thrombosis	0.9–2.3
Wound infection, seroma, dehiscence	0.4–1.7
Lymphocele	0.4–1.4
Rectal injury	0.1–1.3
Prolonged ileus	0.1–1.0
Cardiac arrhythmia	0.3–0.6
Myocardial infarction	0.4
Ureteral injury	0.1–0.3

Autologous blood donation before surgery was popular for some years, but because few patients require transfusion these days, the use of this expensive option has declined.[12] A technique gaining increasing acceptance is intraoperative normovolemic hemodilution. After induction of anesthesia, 2–3 units of blood are removed, the circulating volume is re-established by means of intravenous solutions, and the units are retransfused once blood loss has been controlled.[13]

This technique has also been combined with the preoperative administration of erythropoietin. Erythropoietin (which can be manufactured in large quantities by recombinant DNA technology) helps to return the blood level to normal after surgical bleeding. However, this product should not be used if there is a history of heart or cerebrovascular disease or uncontrolled hypertension.

Thromboembolic complications

Deep venous thrombosis and pulmonary embolism are serious and potentially fatal complications of radical prostatectomy (Table 2).[7–10,14]

Rectal injury

Because of its proximity to the prostate, the rectum can be injured during mobilization of the gland. Fortunately, this occurs only rarely.[7–9,11,15]

Although rectal injury is a serious complication, most cases can be treated by primary repair without temporary colostomy. Some surgeons routinely perform preoperative mechanical and antibiotic bowel prep; others use only a fleet enema on the evening before surgery.

Death

Current surgical and anesthetic techniques and perioperative care are such that radical prostatectomy is a safe procedure, and death related to the surgery is rare. Keetch and collaborators[11] reported no deaths in a series of 810 patients, and Igel and colleagues[8] reported a mortality rate of 0.6%. Reviews of Medicare patients over 65 years of age in the United States have reported 30-day mortality rates ranging from 0.5% to between 1% and 2%,[16,17] and a review of 1059 patients younger than 65 years reported a 30-day mortality rate of 0.28%.[18] Careful selection of patients for this procedure is important and, for those with serious coexisting conditions, the alternatives of radiation therapy or watchful waiting should be considered.

Other complications

The first 12 weeks at home are a time of major adjustment — to both the trauma of the surgery and the challenge of reintegrating into family and work life. Transient physical problems include intermittent bouts of abdominal pain, constipation, diarrhea, incontinence, hematuria and fatigue. Constipation and diarrhea may both be treated effectively by fibre supplements such as bran cereal or psyllium hydrophilic mucilloid.

It is important to perform Kegel exercises to strengthen the external

Table 2: Reported annual incidence of deep venous thrombosis (DVT) and pulmonary embolism (PE) after radical prostatectomy

Reference	Complication; incidence, %	
	DVT	PE
Igel et al[8]	1.2	2.7
Leandri et al[9]	2.3	0.8
Litwiller et al[14] (n = 428)	0.9	0.7
Ramsey et al[7] (n = 878)	1.3	1.7
Walsh[10] (n = 900)	1.0*	1.0*

*Total incidence for either condition was 1%.

urethral sphincter. In addition, the patient should avoid driving a vehicle until the catheter has been removed and should avoid sitting in any one position for too long.

Late complications

Bladder-neck contracture

Scarring may occur at the site of the vesico-urethral anastomosis, which could lead to stricture and bladder-neck contracture. This has been reported in 1.3% to 22% of patients who have undergone radical prostatectomy.[19] Keetch and collaborators[11] reported that this complication occurred in 5% of a series of 810 patients. Among the first 500 patients, the rate was 7.8%, but among the subsequent 310 patients, it was only 0.6%. Surgical technique is obviously important for this complication. Surya and colleagues[19] found that excessive intraoperative blood loss, extravasation of urine at the anastomotic site and a prior transurethral prostatic operation were significant contributing factors to bladder-neck contracture. Treatment involves dilatation of the stricture or urethrotomy performed transurethrally. Care must be taken when performing urethrotomy to prevent damage to the external urinary sphincter, which could result in incontinence.

Urinary incontinence

This is probably the complication most feared by men undergoing radical prostatectomy. Fortunately, the incidence of severe incontinence after contemporary radical prostatectomy is low and, for those unfortunate enough to experience this problem, effective treatment is available. Complete incontinence rates of 0% to 17% and stress incontinence rates of 0% to 35% have been reported.[20] However, improvements in surgical technique have significantly reduced the occurrence of this problem.

Igel and colleagues[8] reported severe to total incontinence in 5% of the patients in their series and mild stress incontinence in 21%. Leandri and associates[9] reported no patients with complete incontinence and only 5% with mild stress incontinence; 90% of those affected had achieved complete urinary control within 6 months after surgery. Keetch and collaborators[11] reported an overall complete continence rate of 94% by 18 months after the operation.

Of the 543 respondents to a questionnaire mailed to all patients who underwent radical prostatectomy in Manitoba between 1985 and 1995, only 3.9% indicated that dripping urine or wetting their pants had been a significant problem; for 7.1%, this had been a moderate problem, for 12.8% a small problem, for 25.5% a very small problem and for 50.7% no problem.[7] No pads were worn by 76.7%, 1 or 2 pads a day were needed by

17.4%, and 3 or more pads per day were needed by 5.4%.

In a review of 593 men who underwent radical prostatectomy, Steiner and associates[20] found that age, mass of the prostate, prior transurethral resection of the prostate, pathologic stage, and preservation or wide excision of the neurovascular bundles had no significant influence on the preservation of urinary control.

Men should be made aware that they will probably be incontinent after the catheter is removed but that control will gradually return over the next few months. Before the surgery, patients should be instructed on how to perform Kegel exercises and should continue these exercises in the postoperative period.

> **KEY POINTS**
> - Urinary incontinence is common in the first few months after surgery, but improvements in surgical techniques have significantly reduced the prevalence of longer-term problems. Incontinence causing significant problems occurs in less than 10% of patients.
> - Erectile dysfunction depends on the age of the patient, preoperative erectile function, the stage of the cancer and the surgical technique.
> - The frequency of loss of erectile function is actually higher than reported in select series from major institutions.
> - Effective treatment options are available for the management of incontinence and erectile dysfunction.

Urinary incontinence as a complication of prostatectomy and the available treatments are discussed in more detail elsewhere in this book.[21]

Erectile dysfunction

With early detection programs, an increasing number of young men are diagnosed with prostate cancer. For these patients in particular preservation of sexual function is important. Before 1982 it was generally assumed that impotence would occur after radical prostatectomy. However, Walsh and Donker[22] showed that the nerves responsible for penile erection lie within the prostatic fascia on the posterolateral border of the prostate. These nerves can be preserved without necessarily compromising the surgeon's ability to eradicate the cancer.[10] Nerve-sparing radical prostatectomy (Fig. 3) has represented a major advance in surgical technique.

How successful is this operation? Walsh[10] reported a postoperative potency rate of 68% among 503 patients, with potency being defined as an erection sufficient for vaginal penetration and orgasm. Younger age, clinically and pathologically confined cancer, and preservation of both neurovascular bundles are associated with a higher rate of postoperative potency. Catalona and Basler[23] have reported preservation of potency after bilateral nerve-sparing surgery in 63% of patients overall and in 75% of patients aged 50–59, 60% of those aged 60–69 and 50% of those 70 years of age and over. The corresponding results for unilateral nerve-sparing surgery were 41% overall and 25%, 48% and 38% for men aged 50–59 years, 60–69 years and 70 years and over respectively.

Unfortunately, the degree of success reported by these authors has not been generally reproducible. In a series from Stanford University, a major referral centre for prostate cancer, only 51 (11.1%) of 459 men who underwent radical prostatectomy maintained erectile function after the procedure.[24] Excluding patients with poor erectile function before surgery, 15.4% of those who underwent unilateral and 35.1% of those who underwent bilateral nerve-sparing prostatectomy remained potent. In that study the patients were asked about their sexual function by an independent observer. A Medicare series using patient-reported results had a similar low potency rate (only 11% of the patients had engaged in unassisted intercourse during the month before questioning).[25] These latter results may partly reflect the older age of the patients in the study (half were older than 70 years at the time of the operation), as well as the fact that the proportion of patients who underwent a nerve-sparing procedure was unknown.

Of 860 patients who underwent radical prostatectomy in Manitoba between 1985 and 1995, 543 (63%) responded to a quality-of-life questionnaire. Of these, 82% claimed that before surgery they had erections firm enough for intercourse, whereas only 10% reported that degree of erection afterward.[7] Although the reported rate of potency before surgery seems high and may reflect patients' failure to recall their erectile function accurately, this value is similar to the 84% reported by Jonler and coworkers.[26]

Geary and colleagues[24] have reported that loss of erectile function after radical prostatectomy does not necessarily mean a loss of erotic sensation or ability to achieve orgasm. However, there will be no significant ejaculation. They reported that, in an informal survey, only 10% of patients (regardless of erectile function) reported decreased orgasmic sensation, 80% reported postoperative orgasms identical with those achieved preoperatively, and 10% reported better orgasms after radical prostatectomy. However, in the Manitoba series,[7] 60% of respondents reported that their ability to reach orgasm was poor (12%) or very poor (47%).

Patients undergoing radical prostatectomy should not be led to expect a 50% or better chance of recovering potency, and men scheduled to have this procedure should be prepared to accept loss of erectile function. For many, this is an acceptable trade-off for the possibility of eradicating the cancer. For others, it represents a major loss. Fortunately, effective treatment options are available to allow most of these men to return to relatively normal sexual activity.

Erectile dysfunction as a complication of prostatectomy and the available treatments are discussed in more detail elsewhere in this book.[21]

Follow-up

A man who undergoes radical prostate surgery should be seen by his surgeon several months after the operation and intermittently for up to 1 year. After that, follow-up may be carried out by the family physician. Depending on the final pathologic assessment, closer, more frequent surveillance may be necessary. At each visit, serum PSA will be measured.

After complete removal of the prostate, the PSA level should drop to undetectable levels, which indicates that all of the cancer cells (and the normal prostate cells) were removed or destroyed. If the PSA level remains detectable within the first year, the odds are that the patient has occult metastatic cancer. A later increase may reflect local recurrence or systemic disease. PSA can indicate a relapse or metastasis many months or even years before the patient has any symptoms or signs of recurrence. Because it may take as long as 7 years or more for recurrence to become evident, a man who has undergone surgery must have yearly examinations indefinitely.

If the pathological findings suggest a high risk of recurrence (e.g., a positive surgical margin, spread to the seminal vesicles or a high Gleason score [over 7]), adjuvant treatment such as radiation therapy to the prostate bed or hormonal therapy may be considered. Results of research on adjuvant treatment are not yet available.

In summary, in the hands of an experienced surgeon, radical prostatectomy offers our patient a high probability of cure with a low risk of incontinence.

References

1. Nam RK, Jewett MAS, Krahn MD. Prostate cancer: 2. Natural history. *CMAJ* 1998;159(6):685-91. [Chapter 2 in this book.]
2. Chodak GW, Thisted RA, Gerber GS, Johansson JE, Adolfsson J, Jones GW, et al. Results of conservative management of clinically localized prostate cancer. *N Engl J Med* 1994;330:242-8.
3. Partin AW, Kattan MW, Subong ENP, Walsh PC, Wojno KJ, Oesterling JE, et al. Combination of prostate-specific antigen, clinical stage, and Gleason score to predict pathological stage of localized prostate cancer. A multi-institutional update. *JAMA* 1997;277:1445-51.
4. Gleave ME, Coupland D, Drachenberg D, Cohen L, Kwong S, Goldenberg SL. Ability of serum prostate-specific antigen levels to predict normal bone scans in patients with newly diagnosed prostate cancer. *Urology* 1996;47:708-12.
5. Goldenberg SL, Klotz LH, Srigley J, Jewett MAS, Mador D, Fradet Y, et al. Randomized, prospective, controlled study comparing radical prostatectomy alone and neoadjuvant androgen withdrawal in the treatment of localized prostate cancer. Canadian Urologic Oncology Group. *J Urol* 1996;156:873-7.
6. Gleave ME, Goldenberg SL, Jones EC, Bruchovsky N, Sullivan LD. Biochemical and pathological effects of 8 months of neoadjuvant androgen withdrawal therapy before radical prostatectomy in patients with clinically confined prostate cancer. *J Urol* 1996;155:213-9.
7. Ramsey EW, Milner J, Casiro M. Quality of life (QL) following radical retropubic prostatectomy. A general population study. *Can J Urol* 1998;45:497A.
8. Igel TC, Barrett DM, Segura JW, Benson RCJ, Rife CC. Perioperative and postoperative complications from bilateral pelvic lymphadenectomy and radical

retropubic prostatectomy. *J Urol* 1987;137:1189-91.
9. Leandri P, Rossignol G, Gauthier JR, Ramon J. Radical retropubic prostatectomy: morbidity and quality of life. Experience with 620 consecutive cases. *J Urol* 1992;147:883-7.
10. Walsh PC. Radical retropubic prostatectomy. In: Walsh PC, Retik AB, Stamey TA, Vaughan ED Jr, editors. *Campbell's urology*. Philadelphia: WB Saunders; 1992. p. 2865-86.
11. Keetch, DW, Andriole GL, Catalona WJ. Complications of radical retropubic prostatectomy. *Am Urol Assoc Update Ser* 1994;13:46-51.
12. Goad JR, Eastham JA, Fitzgerald KB, Kattan MW, Collini MP, Yawn DH, et al. Radical retropubic prostatectomy: limited benefit of autologous blood donation. *J Urol* 1995;154:2103-9.
13. Monk TG, Goodnough LT, Brikmeyer JD, Brecher ME, Catalona WJ. Acute normovolemic hemodilution is a cost-effective alternative to preoperative autologous blood donation by patients undergoing radical retropubic prostatectomy. *Transfusion* 1995;35:559-65.
14. Litwiller SE, Djavan B, Klopukh BV, Richiev JC, Roehrborn CG. Radical retropubic prostatectomy for localized carcinoma of the prostate in a large metropolitan hospital: changing trends over a 10 year period (1984–1994). *Urology* 1995;45:813-22.
15. Borland RN, Walsh PC. The management of rectal injury during radical retropubic prostatectomy. *J Urol* 1992;147:905-7.
16. Lu-Yao GL, McLerran D, Wasson J, Wennberg JE. An assessment of radical prostatectomy. Time trends, geographic variation and outcomes. *JAMA* 1993; 269:2633-6.
17. Mark DH. Mortality of patients after radical prostatectomy: analysis of recent Medicare claims. *J Urol* 1994;152:896-8.
18. Optenberg SA, Wojcik BE, Thompson IM. Morbidity and mortality following radical prostatectomy: a national analysis of Civilian Health and Medical Program of the Uniformed Services beneficiaries. *J Urol* 1995;153:1870-2.
19. Surya BV, Provet J, Johanson KE, Brown J. Anastomotic strictures following radical prostatectomy: risk factors and management. *J Urol* 1990;143:755-8.
20. Steiner MS, Morton RA, Walsh PC. Impact of anatomical radical prostatectomy on urinary continence. *J Urol* 1991;145:512-5.
21. Hassouna MM, Heaton JPW. Prostate cancer: 8. Urinary incontinence and erectile dysfunction. *CMAJ* 1999;160:78-86. [Chapter 8 in this book.]
22. Walsh PC, Donker PJ. Impotence following radical prostatectomy: insight into etiology and prevention. *J Urol* 1982;128:492-7.
23. Catalona WJ, Basler JW. Return of erections and urinary continence following nerve sparing radical retropubic prostatectomy. *J Urol* 1993;150:905-7.
24. Geary ES, Dendinger TE, Freiha FS, Stamey TA. Nerve sparing radical prostatectomy: a different view. *J Urol* 1995;154:145-9.
25. Fowler JE Jr, Barry MJ, Lu-Yao G, Roman A, Wasson J, Wennberg JE. Patient-reported complications and follow-up treatment after radical prostatectomy. The national Medicare experience: 1988–1990 (updated June 1993). *Urology* 1993;42:622-9.
26. Jonler M, Messing EM, Rhodes PR, Bruskewitz RC. Sequelae of radical prostatectomy. *Br J Urol* 1994;74:352-8.

7

Radiation therapy for localized disease

Padraig Warde, MB BCh, BAO; Charles Catton, MD;
Mary K. Gospodarowicz, MD

A 65-year-old man visits his general practitioner for his annual physical examination. On rectal examination the physician discovers a small nodule in the right lobe of his prostate gland. The patient has had no urinary symptoms and is in excellent general health. Sexual function is normal. He has no family history of prostate cancer; his father died of a stroke at age 86 years. The prostate-specific antigen level is elevated (9.3 ng/mL), and transrectal ultrasound-guided biopsy of the nodule reveals adenocarcinoma of the prostate, with a Gleason score of 7. Systematic biopsies of the left lobe yield normal results. At a follow-up visit he tells his physician, "I have been doing some research, and it appears that I should have treatment. However, what is less clear is what form of therapy this should take — surgery or radiation treatment. If radiation, should it be external or interstitial? Please tell me what you can about the state of the art with respect to radiation therapy."

Localized prostate cancer can be treated using potentially curative approaches (e.g., radical prostatectomy and radiation therapy) or palliative approaches with immediate or delayed hormone therapy. Observation or "watchful waiting" is, in essence, a form of delayed therapy, because the disease usually requires treatment in the future. However, in the medical community, there is a lack of consensus regarding the best treatment for patients with localized prostate cancer,[1] especially in terms of the choice between radical prostatectomy and radiation therapy.

This lack of consensus stems from the excellent long-term survival rates among patients with localized disease regardless of treatment approach. No direct comparison of the outcomes of patients treated with surgery and those treated with radiation therapy in a prospective randomized trial is available. The choice of therapy is made by the patient after consultation with a urologist and radiation oncologist; taken into account are the extent of the disease, the tumour grade, the prostate-specific antigen (PSA) level, comorbid conditions and the patient's preference.

Two radiotherapeutic interventions are available to treat localized prostate cancer: external-beam radiation therapy and interstitial brachytherapy. The former uses high-energy linear accelerators and remains the most common approach in most centres. In interstitial brachytherapy, radioactive sources are placed in direct contact with the tumour in the prostate gland as a temporary or permanent implant. The development of improved technology for placement of these implants has recently renewed interest in this approach.[2]

External-beam radiation therapy

Longitudinal multicentre studies have documented excellent long-term overall survival rates among patients with localized prostate cancer treated with external-beam radiation therapy. In one study[3] involving 690 patients with clinically localized disease (T1/T2 N0),[4] the 10-year survival rate was 60%. This rate is similar to the 10-year cause-specific survival rate of 75% reported in an age-matched cohort.[3] Similar results have been reported from many other centres (Table 1).[3,5–8]

Although these results are encouraging, overall survival may not be the most appropriate measure of treatment efficacy in older men with other competing causes of death. Also, cause-specific survival rates can be misleading, because the exact cause of death in elderly people is often difficult to ascertain. The definition of failure following radiation therapy depends on the endpoint measured. For most types of cancer, local

Table 1: Overall and cause-specific survival rates among patients with early-stage (T1 or T2) prostate cancer who underwent external-beam radiation therapy

Study	No. of patients	Tumour stage	5-year survival rate, %		10-year survival rate, %	
			Overall	Cause specific	Overall	Cause specific
Duncan et al[5]	70	T1	83.8	93	57.8	79
	341	T2	81.8	92	53.6	66
Perez et al[6]	48	T1b	85	78	70	60
	252	T2	82	76	65	56
Shipley et al[7]	126	T2	85	–	–	–
Zagars et al[8]	32	T1b	74	90	68	–
	82	T2	93	89	70	85

recurrence or distant metastasis is regarded as evidence of failure. However, for prostate cancer, a tumour marker, PSA, has refined our ability to detect progressive disease. The currently accepted definition of biochemical recurrence is 3 consecutive rising PSA values after PSA level has reached a nadir.[9] With the use of PSA testing to assess treatment outcome, biochemical failure is observed earlier and more frequently than clinical failure. In a cohort of 504 men treated with radiation therapy, the biochemical disease-free survival rate at 10 years was only 40%.[10] Similar results have been reported by others,[3,6] which indicates that, on the basis of a biochemical definition of cure, less than half of the patients treated with radiation therapy in the past have been cured of prostate cancer.

Various strategies to improve treatment results have been proposed, including reducing tumour bulk before radiation therapy with the use of neoadjuvant hormone therapy and increasing the radiation dose to the primary tumour (Table 2). Adding hormone therapy is a more attractive option than increasing the radiation dose, because of the potential to improve local control (without the increased risk of complications from radiation therapy) and to eradicate occult metastatic disease.

Hormone therapy

Neoadjuvant hormone therapy is given *before* definitive treatment such as surgery or radiation therapy; adjuvant hormone therapy is given *after* definitive treatment. Both strategies are used in the management of patients with localized prostate cancer. The mechanisms of action of neoadjuvant hormone therapy include the following:

- It reduces the number of tumour cells, specifically clonogens (tumour stem cells that have the capacity to divide indefinitely), thus making it easier for radiation therapy to eradicate them.
- When combined with radiation therapy it may enhance tumour cell kill in the prostate through a common mechanism of cell death such as apoptosis (an intrinsic cell suicide program under complex genetic regulation).
- It improves the nutritional and oxygenation status of the tumour, thereby increasing the number of cancer cells killed by each fraction of radiation.[11]

In patients with locally advanced pro-

Table 2: Potential strategies to improve results of radiation therapy for localized prostate cancer

Aim	Examples of techniques
Improvement of dose distribution between tumour and normal tissue	Conformal radiotherapy; proton therapy; brachytherapy
Reduction of tumour volume	Neoadjuvant hormone therapy
Improvement in nutritional and oxygenation status of tumour	Neoadjuvant hormone therapy
Biological modification	Altered fractionation; use of radiosensitizers; neutron therapy

> **KEY POINTS**
> - The chances of long-term survival for patients with localized prostate cancer are excellent regardless of treatment.
> - There is no clear difference in outcome between radiation therapy and surgery for patients with localized prostate cancer; the choice will depend on the extent of the disease, comorbid conditions and patient preference.
> - External-beam radiation therapy results in high overall survival rates, but less than half of patients undergoing conventional treatment are likely to be "cured."

state cancer (stage T3 or T4) the role of neoadjuvant and adjuvant hormone therapy has been assessed in prospective randomized trials, and combining radiation therapy with hormone therapy was shown to improve local control and survival. The European Organization for Research and Treatment of Cancer Radiotherapy Group[12] recently reported the results of a study of 415 patients randomly chosen to receive external-beam radiation therapy either alone or with 3 years of adjuvant luteinizing hormone-releasing hormone therapy. With a median follow-up of 45 months the overall 5-year survival rate was 79% in the combined treatment group, as compared with 62% in the radiation-only group ($p = 0.001$). Improvement was also seen in disease-free survival and local tumour control. The 5-year PSA progression-free rate was 81% in the combined treatment group and 43% in the radiation-only group. This trial confirmed the superiority of combined treatment in locally advanced disease. Other studies, such as the Radiation Therapy Oncology Group trial 86-10, have shown some benefit with neoadjuvant hormone therapy in terms of local control and disease-free survival in locally advanced prostate cancer.[13,14] However, no improvement in overall survival has been shown in any study of neoadjuvant hormone therapy. The timing and duration of neoadjuvant and adjuvant hormone therapy in locally advanced prostate cancer remain unclear and are being addressed in ongoing trials.

Current studies are addressing the role of neoadjuvant and adjuvant hormone therapy in patients with early-stage prostate cancer (T1 and T2). At present the routine use of neoadjuvant or adjuvant hormone therapy in these patients is considered experimental. Neoadjuvant treatment, usually chemotherapy, in other cancers has not been shown to be of benefit. Neoadjuvant treatment could potentially be detrimental by delaying definitive therapy or by stimulating repopulation of surviving tumour cells, making subsequent radiation therapy less effective. However, these largely theoretical concerns have not been supported by clinical data.

Increasing the radiation dose

Another strategy for improving the effect of external-beam radiation therapy is to increase the radiation dose using conformal techniques. Advances in computer technology have allowed the development of 3-dimensional conformal radiation therapy and the delivery of high-precision radiation therapy. Currently, satisfactory techniques are available to deliver radiotherapy in a manner that moulds the spatial distribution of the dose to the precise 3-dimensional configuration of the prostate. These techniques also minimize the exposure to radiation of the surrounding structures.

> **KEY POINTS**
> - Results of external-beam radiation therapy may be improved by increasing the dose using conformal techniques or by using neoadjuvant hormone therapy.
> - Interstitial brachytherapy — placement of a radioactive source in the prostate in direct contact with the tumour — is a reasonable alternative to surgery or external beam radiation therapy in patients with early-stage, low-grade disease.

Retrospective studies have suggested that doses of 70 Gy or more improve local tumour control and biochemical freedom from relapse.[15] Increasing the radiation dose can be done safely provided the distribution of radiation between the prostate and surrounding normal tissues (particularly the bladder and rectum) is optimized using conformal techniques.

When these conformal techniques were used in a consecutive series of 202 patients with early-stage (T1c) prostate cancer[16] the 5-year rate for biochemical freedom from relapse was 97% among patients with pretreatment PSA levels of less than 10 ng/mL and 88% among those with pretreatment levels of 10–20 ng/mL. Less than 1% of patients had severe rectal or urinary sequelae, and 61% maintained sexual potency. However, chronic rectal bleeding can occur after escalated-dose radiation therapy; it may require ongoing treatment and can significantly affect a patient's quality of life.[17] Similar data on biochemical freedom from disease have been reported from other centres using dose-escalation protocols, and overall these results are comparable to those from recent reports of nerve-sparing radical prostatectomy.[18,19]

An even more refined delivery method is intensity-modulated radiation therapy. This form of treatment involves the production of a conformal radiation field by a moving multileaf collimator and accelerator gantry. During treatment, a non-uniform radiation dose is delivered to the patient from various entry points, allowing for a uniform dose distribution within the tumour while preventing exposure of normal tissues to a high dose. This technique is now being introduced into clinical practice, and early results are promising for the treatment of localized prostate cancer.[20]

Although the initial experience with dose-escalation radiation therapy provides reasons for optimism, the long-term benefits for patients with localized prostate cancer await assessment in phase III randomized trials. The Radiation Therapy Oncology Group is currently embarking on such a study.

Interstitial brachytherapy

Interstitial brachytherapy using iodine 125 was extensively used in the management of localized prostate cancer in the late 1970s and early 1980s. The initial results were excellent, and serious side effects were rare. In particular, impotence rates were believed to be much lower than those seen with external-beam radiation therapy. However, the long-term results were disappointing, and the technique was abandoned. In retrospect, the poor results were likely related to imprecise implantation techniques. Accurate placement of radioactive sources is required to deliver a uniform radiation dose to the whole prostate gland. Early treatments relied on free-hand placement of the radioactive sources, which resulted in dose distributions that were not homogeneous because of less than ideal positioning of the radioactive sources.[21]

Recently, the use of transrectal ultrasonography and computed tomography to direct transperineal implantation has resulted in much improved clinical outcomes.[22] These techniques allow for a more uniform placement of the radioactive sources and, consequently, improved dose distribution.

The radiation dose delivered by brachytherapy using ^{125}I implants is substantially greater than that delivered by external-beam radiation therapy. Recent studies involving patients with a PSA level of less than 10 ng/mL showed results similar to those achieved with external-beam dose-escalation protocols, with more than 85% of patients biochemically free of disease at 3 years.[22,23]

The morbidity profile of brachytherapy in terms of acute reactions is favourable. Treatment involves an outpatient procedure with minimal intraoperative complications. Symptoms of increased frequency of urination and urgency are common but are usually mild and self-limiting. Few patients require temporary catheterization to alleviate bladder outlet obstruction.

However, late treatment complications are of greater concern. A recent report of 92 patients documented persistent moderately severe urinary symptoms 2 years after implantation in 14 patients and radiation-induced rectal ulceration in 5 patients.[24] The incidence of complications was considerably lower among those who had not had transurethral resection of the prostate in the past. Preliminary data on impotence in men managed with seed implantation indicate preservation of erectile function in the majority of patients.[25]

To improve these techniques further, newer isotopes, including palladium 103 and iridium 192, have recently been introduced into clinical practice. ^{103}Pd has a higher dose rate than ^{125}I and, although the clinical significance of this is controversial, mathematical models suggest that ^{125}I would be better in the treatment of slower-growing tumours and ^{103}Pd would be more effective for rapidly growing tumours.[2] Currently, ^{125}I is used primarily for well- to moderately differentiated tumours (Gleason score 2–6), and ^{103}Pd is used in patients with poorly differentiated tumours (Gleason score 7–10). ^{192}Ir is used in temporary seed implantation and, because of a significant high-energy gamma radiation component, requires sophisticated shielding for medical personnel. In contrast, both ^{103}Pd and ^{125}I produce only low-energy gamma radiation, and protection for medical personnel and patients' families is relatively easy. There is general agreement that the optimal candidates for permanent seed implantation are patients with stage T1 or T2 tumours with low-grade disease (Gleason score ≤ 6) and a PSA level of 10 ng/mL or less. Comparison of treatment outcomes with surgery and external-beam radiation therapy suggests that brachytherapy is as efficacious in terms of PSA progression-free survival in this group of patients.[26] However, long-term results with brachytherapy are not available, and randomized clinical trials are necessary to delineate its role in prostate cancer management.

Complications of external-beam radiation therapy

As with any curative cancer therapy, radiation therapy commonly results in minor complications but rarely in major ones. Unlike surgery, though, this treatment does not require admission to hospital, and there are few contraindications to its use. Side effects may occur as acute reactions during and immediately after radiation treatment and as late reactions that may become apparent within several months or even 3 to 10 years after treatment.

Acute reactions

Acute reactions are due to specific injury of mucosal epithelium within the irradiated volume and to nonspecific factors such as fatigue. The onset of symptoms (Table 3) depends on the number of weeks over which the radiation is given and on the turnover rate of epithelial cells. For conventional prostatic irradiation given over 6–7 weeks, symptoms usually develop 2–3 weeks after treatment starts, peak at 5–6 weeks and begin to subside toward the completion of treatment, when re-epithelialization begins.

The severity of the reaction depends on the total radiation dose given and the

Table 3: Symptoms of acute complications of radiation therapy for localized prostate cancer

Common
Fatigue
Frequency, urgency, dysuria, nocturia
Rectal tenesmus, mucous discharge and frequent, pellet-like stools
Diarrhea

Uncommon
Urinary retention due to prostatic edema (usually an exacerbation of pre-existing bladder outlet obstruction)
Rectal bleeding

time over which it is given, the volume of mucosa in the treatment area and the patient's inherent sensitivity to radiation. The tissues commonly at risk are in the prostate itself, at the base of the bladder and in the anterior rectal wall; they may also include the small bowel if prophylactic nodal irradiation is used.

In a series of 914 patients treated with curative radiation therapy 24% experienced genitourinary symptoms and 43% had gastrointestinal side effects.[27] Most of the reactions were minor. Severe acute genitourinary or gastrointestinal sequelae that require a halt in therapy are uncommon; such effects were identified in 2.5% of all treated patients in another large series.[6]

Late reactions

Late reactions (Table 4) result from connective-tissue injury that develops months to years after therapy. Typically, progressive microvascular injury produces subepithelial telangiectasia and fibrosis in the submucosal layer and muscular layer of the organ wall, which in turn lead to a more fragile mucosa that has a tendency to minor bleeding, along with a degree of chronic functional change. This fibrosis rarely disrupts the microvasculature to the point where chronic mucosal ulceration and necrosis may result. The severity of a late reaction depends mainly on the total

Table 4: Late complications of radiation therapy for localized prostate cancer

Complication	Treatment
Rectum	
Mild: Intermittent, mild rectal bleeding; change in bowel habits not requiring medication	None required
Moderate: Chronic rectal irritation and mucous discharge requiring medication; persistent rectal bleeding	Steroid suppositories or foam retention enemas; sulfasalazine
Severe: Rectal ulceration (very rare)	Defunctioning colostomy
Bladder	
Mild: Mild increase in urinary frequency or nocturia	None required
Moderate: Frequency or nocturia requiring medication; intermittent hematuria	Antispasmodics; coagulation of bleeding telangiectasia
Severe: Contracted bladder with capacity less than 100 mL; chronic hematuria (very rare)	Urinary diversion
Incontinence	
Rare; almost always associated with TURP before or after radiation	Artificial sphincter
Urethral stricture and bladder-neck contracture	
Rare; often associated with TURP before radiation	Urethral dilatation
Prostate	
Loss of seminal fluid with scanty or dry ejaculate	None available
Erectile dysfunction	
Incomplete or complete dysfunction in 50% of patients; believed due to microvascular injury to branches of internal pudendal and penile arteries	Medical: sildenafil (Viagra); intracorporeal injection of papavarine Mechanical: vacuum pump; surgical implants
Leg and genital edema	
Rare; almost always associated with prior pelvic node dissection	Compression stockings; compression pump

Note: TURP = transurethral resection of prostate.

radiation dose given, the size of the daily radiation fraction given and the amount of sensitive normal tissue in the treatment volume. The severity of an acute reaction does not predict the severity of any late reaction that might occur. Severe late reactions often improve over time, but unlike acute reactions they may never completely resolve. Modern treatment techniques are designed to minimize the risk of severe late reactions.

The risk of a late reaction becoming permanent is of greater concern to patients than the risk of an acute reaction. Fortunately, apart from sexual impotence, severe late genitourinary and gastrointestinal complications rarely follow conventional curative radiation therapy for prostate cancer. A large multicentre study has identified that severe late complications occur in less than 2% of patients.[28]

Risks of late reactions

Our understanding of the risks of complications from prostatic radiation therapy is based on data collected retrospectively and prospectively using toxicity grading systems like the Radiation Therapy Oncology Group toxicity score,[29] which grades treatment-related side effects from the physician's perspective. Grading tools that determine the impact of treatment-related side effects on quality of life from the patient's perspective are now in use, but data from them are limited.[28]

The combined results of large series of curative treatment in a total of 2216 men with prostate cancer showed that the risk of proctitis with rectal bleeding after radiation therapy ranged from 2.6% to 14.9% and persisted for more than 6 months in less than 3% of patients.[30] The risk of persistent diarrhea requiring medication was 2.1%. Similarly, cystitis with hematuria occurred in 2.6% to 10.8% of treated patients and persisted for more than 6 months in less than 3%. Urethral stricture or bladder-neck contracture that could not be corrected by simple endoscopic procedures was reported in 1.1% of cases. Urinary incontinence, a rare complication of prostatic radiation therapy, was reported in only 0.9% of cases. A history of transurethral resection of the prostate before or after radiation therapy may be a major risk factor for this complication.[30]

A dry ejaculate is a common late side effect of mucosal injury due to prostatic irradiation. Permanent sexual impotence is also a common side effect and is of more significance to patients. The actual risk of impotence secondary to prostatic irradiation is not precisely known, because the causes are multifactorial among the predominantly elderly men with prostate cancer who undergo radiation therapy. It is widely accepted that about 50% of all previously potent men will become impotent within 5 years after curative prostatic irradiation.[27] The risk of impotence is higher among older men with borderline pretreatment erectile function than among younger and healthier men.

Leg and genital edema are rare complications and are usually related to a previous pelvic node dissection. Radionecrosis of pelvic bones is a serious but extremely rare complication and is almost never seen with modern treatment techniques unless an error in treatment prescription or radiation delivery has occurred.

Minimizing the risk of complications

Careful treatment planning and modern delivery systems will minimize the risk of serious radiation injuries.[31] To reduce the risk of incontinence or stricture, transurethral resection of the bladder neck should be avoided in patients who are about to undergo or who have received prostatic irradiation.

Patients with large-volume glands who require a larger radiation volume are at higher risk of moderate or severe acute and late rectal injury.[32] Patients with pre-existing symptoms of bladder outlet obstruction are more likely to have increased obstructive symptoms after radiation therapy. In both cases, reduction of prostate bulk with hormone therapy may lessen the risk of severe complications.

There is no proven method for reducing the risk of erectile dysfunction following radiation therapy, but newer methods of treatment such as 3-dimensional conformal radiation therapy and low-dose-rate brachytherapy protect more of the normal rectal and bladder wall from the high-dose radiation and may further reduce the risk of moderate and severe reactions.

Management of complications

Acute reactions

Mild to moderate acute reactions are managed symptomatically. Local measures, including sitz baths, cortisone cream and suppositories, reduce the symptoms of acute treatment-related proctitis. Antispasmodics and urinary analgesics (e.g., phenazopyridine [pyridium]) will treat mild to moderate cystitis and urethritis. Urinary retention is rare and, when present, requires catheterization; radiation therapy can proceed with a catheter in place. Severe bladder or rectal symptoms are extremely uncommon and may require a break in or premature cessation of radiation therapy.

Late reactions

A slight change in bowel or bladder habits or mild intermittent and painless rectal bleeding requires no specific therapy. Such bleeding usually occurs with the passing of stools and its cause must be differentiated from treatment-related proctitis. Proctoscopy of a patient with proctitis will typically demonstrate a friable mucosa with telangiectasia, and these changes are usually most prominent on the anterior rectal wall adjacent to the prostate.

Bleeding from proctitis must not be mistaken for hemorrhoidal bleeding; inappropriate hemorrhoidal surgery after prostatic irradiation leads to poor healing and anal stricture. Coincident hemorrhoids should be managed medically.

Persistent rectal symptoms must be investigated and other causes ruled out. Treatment-related proctitis responds to anti-inflammatory drugs such as cortisone in foam retention enemas twice daily for 2 weeks or sulfasalazine (Salazopyrin) for longer-term therapy. The use of short-chain fatty acid enemas in the treatment of proctitis after radiation therapy is currently under investigation and may prove useful.

> **KEY POINTS**
> - Radiation therapy commonly results in minor side effects but rarely in major ones. Unlike surgery, though, this treatment does not require admission to hospital, and there are few contraindications to its use.
> - Common acute reactions to radiation therapy are fatigue, frequent and urgent urination, rectal tenesmus and diarrhea. These often begin a few weeks after treatment starts, but they subside after the completion of treatment.
> - Late reactions, resulting from connective-tissue injury, develop months to years after therapy but occur in less than 2% of patients.

The development of microscopic or overt hematuria following treatment requires investigation to rule out other causes. Treatment-related cystitis can be diagnosed only using cystoscopy to identify radiation-induced bladder changes. Chronic bladder irritation from radiation-induced cystitis may require long-term therapy with antispasmodics, and persistent hematuria may require coagulation of bleeding telangiectasia. In very severe cases, persistent rectal or bladder symptoms may ultimately require surgical urinary or rectal diversion. Impotence, when present, will become apparent 18 to 60 months after radiation therapy and may be managed with intracorporeal therapy or mechanical aids.

Comments

Radiation therapy is an effective treatment option for patients with localized prostate cancer. The Prostate Cancer Clinical Guidelines Panel of the American Urological Association has concluded that outcomes data are inadequate for valid comparison of treatments because of large differences among treatment groups in such significant characteristics as age, tumour grade and pelvic lymph node status.[33] The panel recommended that patients with newly diagnosed, clinically localized prostate cancer should be informed of all available treatment options and that they should take part in formulating the treatment decision. Radiation therapy is contraindicated in patients with inflammatory bowel disease and those previously treated with radiation therapy (e.g., for seminoma).

Patients with early-stage disease (T1b–T2a with a Gleason score of 7 or less and a PSA level of 10 ng/mL or less), such as the man described at the beginning of this chapter, can be treated successfully with either external-beam radiation therapy or interstitial brachytherapy. Patients with more advanced disease (a higher PSA level, larger tumour size or higher Gleason score) should be considered for escalated-dose conformal radiation therapy or combined radiation therapy and hormone therapy.

Large prospective randomized phase III trials should be instituted to address the issue of optimal therapy. It is somewhat disheartening that in 1990 only 1.7% of men with prostate cancer in the United States were enrolled in a clinical trial. Only continued research and properly designed randomized trials will define the optimal management of patients with localized prostate cancer.

Trends in radiotherapy are also discussed by Trachtenberg and associates elsewhere in this book.[34]

References

1. Moore M, O'Sullivan B, Tannock I. How expert physicians would wish to be treated if they had genitourinary cancer. *J Clin Oncol* 1988;6:1736-45.
2. Grimm P, Blasko J, Ragde H, Sylvester J, Clarke C. Does brachytherapy have a role in the treatment of prostate cancer? *Hematol Oncol Clin North Am* 1996;10:653-90.
3. Bagshaw M, Cox R, Hancock S. Control of prostate cancer with radiotherapy: long-term results. *J Urol* 1994;152:1781-5.
4. Sobin LH, Wittekind C, editors. *TNM classification of malignant tumours*. 5th ed. New York: Wiley-Liss, Inc; 1997.
5. Duncan W, Warde P, Catton C, Munro A, Lakier R, Gadalla T, et al. Carcinoma of the prostate: results of radical radiotherapy (1970–1985). *Int J Radiat Oncol Biol Phys* 1993;26:203-10.
6. Perez C, Hanks G, Leibel S, Zietman A, Fuks Z, Lee W. Localized carcinoma of the prostate (stages T1b, T1c, T2 and T3): review of management with external beam radiation therapy. *Cancer* 1993;72:3156-73.
7. Shipley W, Prout G, Coachman N, McManus P, Healey E. Radiation therapy for localized prostate cancer: experience at the Massachusetts General Hospital (1973–1981). *J Natl Cancer Inst Monogr* 1988;7:67-73.
8. Zagars G, von Eschenbach A, Johnson D, Oswald M. The role of radiation therapy in stages A2 and B adenocarcinoma of the prostate. *Int J Radiat Oncol Biol Phys* 1988;14:701-9.
9. American Society for Therapeutic Radiology and Oncology Consensus Panel. Consensus statement: guidelines for PSA following radiation therapy. *Int J Radiat Oncol Biol Phys* 1997;37:1035-41.
10. Zietman A, Coen J, Dallow K, Shipley W. The treatment of prostate cancer by conventional radiation therapy: an analysis of long-term outcome. *Int J Radiat Oncol Biol Phys* 1995;32:287-92.

11. Zietman A, Prince E, Nakfoor B, Shipley W. Neoadjuvant androgen suppression with radiation in the management of locally advanced adenocarcinoma of the prostate: experimental and clinical results. *Urology* 1997;49:74-83.
12. Bolla M, Gonzalez D, Warde P, Dubois J, Mirimanoff R, Storme G, et al. Improved survival in patients with locally advanced prostate cancer treated with radiotherapy and goserelin. *N Engl J Med* 1997;337:295-300.
13. Pilepich M, Winter K, Roach M, Russell A, Sause W, Rubin P, et al. Phase III Radiation Therapy Oncology Group (RTOG) trial 86-10 of androgen deprivation before and during radiotherapy in locally advanced carcinoma of the prostate [abstract A1185]. *Proc ASCO* 1998;17:308a.
14. Laverdiere J, Gomez JL, Cusan L, Suburu ER, Diamond P, Lemay M, et al. Beneficial effect of combination hormonal therapy administered prior and following external beam radiation therapy in localized prostate cancer. *Int J Radiat Oncol Biol Phys* 1997;37:247-52.
15. Pollack A, Zagars G. External beam radiotherapy dose response of prostate cancer. *Int J Radiat Oncol Biol Phys* 1997;39:1011-8.
16. Hanks G, Hanlon A, Pinover W, Al-Saleem T, Schultheiss T. Radiation therapy as treatment for stage T1c prostate cancers. *World J Urol* 1997;15:369-72.
17. Teshima T, Hanks G, Hanlon A, Peter R, Schultheiss T. Rectal bleeding after conformal 3D treatment of prostate cancer: time to occurrence, response to treatment and duration of morbidity. *Int J Radiat Oncol Biol Phys* 1997;39:77-83.
18. Zelefsky MJ, Leibel SA, Gaudin PB, Kutcher GJ, Fleshner NE, Venkatramen ES, et al. Dose escalation with three-dimensional conformal radiation therapy affects the outcome in prostate cancer. *Int J Radiat Oncol Biol Phys* 1998;41:491-500.
19. D'Amico AV, Whittington R, Kaplan I, Beard C, Jiroutek M, Malkowicz SB, et al. Equivalent biochemical failure-free survival after external beam radiation therapy or radical prostatectomy in patients with a pretreatment prostate specific antigen of < 4–20 ng/ml. *Int J Radiat Oncol Biol Phys* 1997;37:1053-8.
20. Reinstein L, Wang X, Burman C, Chen Z, Mohan R, Kutcher G, et al. A feasibility study of automated inverse treatment planning for cancer of the prostate. *Int J Radiat Oncol Biol Phys* 1998;40:207-14.
21. Porter A, Blasko J, Grimm P, Reddy S, Ragde H. Brachytherapy for prostate cancer. *CA Cancer J Clin* 1995;45:165-78.
22. Ragde H, Blasko J, Grimm P, Kenny G, Sylvester J, Hoak D, et al. Brachytherapy for clinically localized prostate cancer: results at 7- and 8-year follow-up. *Semin Surg Oncol* 1997;13:438-43.
23. D'Amico A, Coleman C. Role of interstitial radiotherapy in the management of clinically organ-confined prostate cancer: the jury is still out. *J Clin Oncol* 1996;14:304-15.
24. Wallner K, Roy J, Harrison L. Tumor control and morbidity following transperineal iodine 125 implantation for stage T1/T2 prostatic carcinoma. *J Clin Oncol* 1996;14:449-53.
25. Stock R, Stone N, Iannuzzi C. Sexual potency following interactive ultrasound-guided brachytherapy for prostate cancer. *Int J Radiat Oncol Biol Phys* 1996;35:267-72.
26. D'Amico AV, Whittington R, Malkowicz SB, Schultz D, Blank K, Broderick GA, et al. Biochemical outcome after radical prostatectomy, external beam radiation therapy, or interstitial radiation therapy for clinically localized prostate cancer. *JAMA* 1998;280:969-74.
27. Bagshaw M, Cox R, Ray G. Status of radiation treatment of prostatic cancer at Stanford University. *J Natl Cancer Inst Monogr* 1988;7:47-51.
28. Beard C, Propert K, Reiker P, Clark J, Kaplan I, Kantoff P, et al. Complications after

treatment with external beam irradiation in early-stage prostate cancer patients: a prospective multiinstitutional outcomes study. *J Clin Oncol* 1997;15:223-30.
29. Perez C, Brady L, editors. *Principles and practice of radiation oncology.* 2nd ed. Philadelphia: JB Lippincott; 1992. p. 51-5.
30. Shipley W, Zietman A, Hanks G, Coen J, Caplan R, Won M, et al. Treatment related sequelae following external beam radiation for prostate cancer: a review with an update in patients with stages T1 and T2 tumor. *J Urol* 1994;152:1799-805.
31. Perez C, Lee H, Anastasios G, Lockett M. Technical factors affecting morbidity in definitive irradiation for localized carcinoma of the prostate. *Int J Radiat Oncol Biol Phys* 1994;28:811-8.
32. Benk V, Adams J, Shipley W, Urie M, McManus P, Efird J, et al. Late rectal bleeding following combined x–ray and proton high dose irradiation for stages T3–T4 prostate cancer. *Int J Radiat Oncol Biol Phys* 1993;26:551-7.
33. Middleton R, Thompson I, Austenfeld M, Cooner W, Correa R, Gibbons R, et al. Prostate Cancer Clinical Guidelines Panel summary report on the management of clinically localized prostate cancer. *J Urol* 1995;154:2144-8.
34. Trachtenberg J, Crook J, Tannock IF. Prostate cancer: 11. Alternative approaches and the future of treatment. *CMAJ* 1999;160:528-34. [Chapter 11 in this book.]

8

Urinary incontinence and erectile dysfunction

Magdy M. Hassouna, MD, PhD; Jeremy P.W. Heaton, MA, MD

A 68-year-old sexually active man is referred to a urologist for consideration of radical prostatectomy following diagnosis of prostate cancer. Rectal examination has revealed a single nodule confined to the prostate, and the Gleason score is 6. The patient has talked to friends and has done some reading and is very concerned about the possibility of urinary incontinence and erectile dysfunction after the surgery.

EDITORS' NOTE: Earlier chapters in this book, those on surgical treatment[1] and radiation therapy,[2] have covered the complications of these treatments. However, because urinary incontinence and erectile dysfunction are such important problems, in terms of both their frequency and their effects on patients' quality of life, we felt that they merit more detailed discussion. Separate sections on these common side effects of radiation therapy and prostatectomy make up the eighth chapter of the book.

Urinary incontinence*

The age-adjusted rate of radical prostatectomy increased almost 6-fold between 1984 and 1990.[3] At the same time as the number of procedures is increasing, surgeons are acquiring more expertise in maintaining the continence mechanism without compromising the surgical goal of extirpating the localized cancer.

---

*This section by Dr. Magdy M. Hassouna.

The apical dissection of the prostate remains the key issue. Some surgeons prefer limited dissection of the puboprostatic ligaments.[4] Others advocate dissection of the preprostatic vein plexus and placement of traction sutures in the urethral stump early in the procedure. With the preservation of the bladder neck[5] and retention of the normal anatomic structure of the sphincteric mechanisms and their nerve supplies, the prevalence of return of continence after radical prostatectomy is now approaching 70% at 1 year after surgery.[6]

Anatomic structure of the bladder outlet

Because of the location of the gland, prostatic surgery necessarily affects the structures that regulate continence. Thus, knowledge of the anatomic structure of the bladder outlet is essential to an understanding of the continence mechanisms.

The inferolateral surfaces of the prostate are related to the anterior parts of the levator ani muscle (Fig. 1). The apex of the prostate is directed toward the external sphincter complex (consisting of the sphincter urethrae and transversus perinei profundus muscles), and the anterior surface of the prostate is connected to the pubic bones by condensation of the pelvic fascia, called the puboprostatic ligaments. The urethra emerges from the surface a little above and in front of the apex. It is important to locate these anatomic landmarks during surgical removal of the prostate.

The external sphincter complex is composed of external and internal skeletal muscle fibres. The external fibres arise from the transverse perineal ligament and sweep backward on both sides of the urethra. The deep (rhabdosphincter) fibres encircle and blend into the wall of the urethra

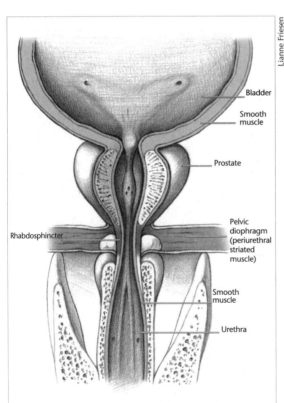

Fig. 1: Anatomy of the pelvic diaphragm.

and extend upward to blend into the capsule of the prostate.[7] Transurethral ultrasonography has revealed that the rhabdosphincter is a vertical structure extending from the membranous urethra to the bladder neck. It does not form a complete collar around the membranous urethra but is shaped like the letter C.[8]

The external sphincter complex is innervated through branches of the pudendal nerves. There is some evidence[9] that part of the somatic innervation to the sphincter is located close to the apex of the prostate.

The bladder and its outlet are involved in the storage and evacuation (voiding) of urine. During the storage phase, the bladder should display good compliance, lack of uninhibited detrusor contractions and a competent outlet that sustains a pressure of at least 40 cm H_2O. The voiding phase involves the relaxation of the pelvic floor, funnelling of the bladder outlet and sustained contraction of the detrusor muscle.

Prevalence of post-prostatectomy urinary incontinence

Urinary incontinence after radical prostatectomy for localized cancer has been the subject of scrutiny in recent years. Questionnaires specific for continence history have revealed that 30% of patients experience some form of urinary incontinence after radical prostatectomy.[6] Other studies have shown that incontinence depends on time since surgery: only 23% of patients are continent after 1 month, but by 12 months 84% to 95% have regained continence.[10–12]

Types of incontinence

Most authors agree that incontinence after radical prostatic surgery is caused by direct damage to the sphincter. Outlet resistance is significantly decreased after radical surgery, as indicated by values for Valsalva leak pressure point (the pressure at which urinary leakage occurs when the person increases abdominal pressure), maximum urethral pressure and functional urethral length. However, outlet resistance increases with time and coincides with regaining of continence.[13,14]

Detrusor instability — the development of unwanted detrusor contraction exceeding 15 cm H_2O during the filling of the bladder — is responsible for incontinence in 41% of patients after surgery.[12,15] A combination of detrusor instability and sphincteric incontinence was found in 52% of patients in another study.[16] Detrusor instability is an important factor in treatment, because in patients with this problem incontinence responds less favourably to techniques to increase outlet resistance than in patients with other causes of incontinence.

Diagnosis

History

The physician should identify the degree and type of incontinence, as well as the time of onset. The number of protective pads used per day by a patient gives an accurate assessment of degree of incontinence. Most patients experience some incontinence after removal of the catheter. Continence gradually improves with time, as evidenced by a continuous decline in the number of protective pads needed. This type of incontinence is usually easy for the patient to describe.

Most patients experience urinary leakage during stressful events such as coughing, stooping and lifting heavy objects. In this situation it is important to assess the patient's normal level of physical activity before starting treatment and to tailor the treatment to the level of activity. For example, patients who have been sedentary may experience more incontinence than they otherwise would if they try to become more physically active after their surgery. Some patients experience urinary leakage associated with a sense of urgency. This should point to the possibility of detrusor instability as a cause of the incontinence.

Urodynamic study

Fluoroscopy remains the standard for diagnosing incontinence. A test is conducted with the patient sitting in front of a fluoroscope. While the bladder is filled with a radiocontrasting substance, intravesicle and intra-abdominal pressures are recorded. The operator is able to visualize the contours of the bladder and pays special attention to the bladder outlet (Fig. 2). Persistent funnelling of the latter denotes incompetence of the

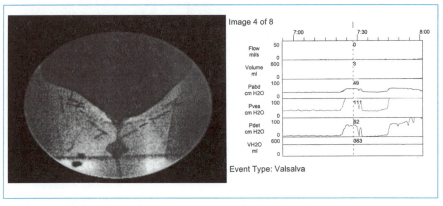

Fig. 2: Fluoroscopy of the bladder and outlet during a Valsalva manoeuvre, with readings for flow and volume of urine; abdominal, vesicular and detrusor pressure; and volume of water in the bladder. Peak actual values of the variables are presented. The horizontal scale is time, in minutes.

sphincteric mechanism. When the bladder is filled to capacity, the patient is asked to perform a Valsalva manoeuvre. Most urodynamic devices allow simultaneous recording of intra-abdominal pressure and fluoroscopic visualization of the bladder outlet. The Valsalva leak pressure point is the pressure at which contrast material seeps through the bladder outlet. A value below 40 cm H_2O denotes a severely incompetent sphincter. During the filling phase, the operator should look for detrusor instability, as evidenced by uninhibited detrusor contraction. Occasionally funnelling of the bladder outlet may be seen during this uninhibited contraction.

> **KEY POINTS**
> - Improvements in surgical techniques have resulted in a rate of continence after radical prostatectomy of 70% (at 1 year after surgery).
> - Incontinence after radical prostatectomy may be caused by direct damage to the sphincter, or it may result from instability of the detrusor muscle.

Treatment

The treatment of urinary incontinence after radical prostatectomy depends on the nature of the mechanism of incontinence.

Pharmacotherapy

The treatment of bladder instability depends greatly on the use of the anticholinergic group of drugs. Oxybutynin remains the standard with which other anticholinergics are compared. The normal dose is 5 mg, taken orally, 3 or 4 times a day, depending on the patient's tolerance of the side effects. The major side effects are dryness of the mucous membranes (which appears in the form of dry throat and conjunctiva as well as constipation) and could precipitate angle-closure glaucoma. Some patients can take oxybutynin on an as-needed basis, which reduces the risk of side effects.

Other anticholinergics — imipramine, flavoxate, propantheline and tolteridine — are less effective, but they have fewer side effects than oxybutynin. Tolteridine has recently been released in Canada as Detrol; this agent can be titrated in increasing doses as it is associated with less dryness of the mouth.

Pelvic floor rehabilitation

Pelvic floor stimulation and biofeedback have been used in rehabilitating the pelvic floor and helping patients regain continence.[17] Treatment consists of several visits (once or twice a week) in which the patient is taught to carry out a series of rapid and sustained pelvic contractions. The intensity of the contractions is monitored by means of an instrument display visible to the patient.

The set-up requires experienced personnel and motivated patients, but this behavioural therapy was successful in restoring continence in 40% to 70% of men in one study.[17] A good response can be expected in patients whose incontinence is due to mild or moderate sphincteric weakness. The results are less favourable for patients who have undergone radiotherapy after radical surgery, because in these patients the musculature of the pelvic floor becomes more fibrotic and less amenable to voluntary contraction.

Endoscopic injection of bulking material

Several bulking agents — among them polytetrafluoroethylene (Teflon), autologous fat and silicone — have been used to augment outlet resistance and thus improve continence. Teflon and silicone were associated with a high rate of migration and granuloma formation, and autologous fat often resulted in poor graft survival and rapid absorption. These bulking agents are not currently in use.

Favourable results have been achieved with bovine collagen cross-linked with glutaraldehyde in patients who are not allergic to the collagen. This substance is injected in either an antegrade or a retrograde manner around the bladder neck and the anastomotic line by means of a cystoscope. The retrograde technique (which involves transurethral injection) has been less successful, mainly because of the poorly developed submucosal spaces that accommodate the injected collagen. These spaces are usually obliterated by the fibrosis that occurs at the anastomotic line. Moreover, the amount of collagen that must be injected has made this approach uneconomical. With the antegrade technique, which uses a flexible cystoscope inserted suprapubically, the collagen is introduced around the bladder neck, where the submucosal space has greater capacity. Although this procedure is more invasive, a short-term study found that the success rate in terms of significant improvement in continence or complete cure was 70%.[18]

Artificial urinary sphincter

The artificial urinary sphincter is another method of treating urinary incontinence after radical prostatectomy. This device has been updated since its original inception in the mid-1970s. The AMS 800 (American Medical System, Guelph, Ont.), the artificial sphincter in current use,[19] consists of a cuff that ranges from 4 to 6 cm in length, a pressure-regulating reservoir and a pump. The cuff is implanted around the bulbar urethra, which is easily accessible through the perineum. Implantation of the cuff around the bladder neck is not usually recommended, since the task of dissecting the planes after such extensive pelvic surgery is formidable.

The reservoir comes in 3 pressure ranges: 50–61, 60–71 and 70–81 cm H_2O. The appropriate pressure depends on the level of physical activity of the patient. However, an unnecessarily elevated pressure can result in pressure necrosis in the urethra and eventual erosion of the cuff. The pressure-regulated reservoir is usually implanted in the prevesical space. However, this placement may be difficult if extensive fibrosis develops after surgery. The pump, which regulates the opening and closing of the cuff, is implanted in the scrotum in a place that is easily accessible to the patient. The side chosen depends on the patient's manual dexterity.

> **KEY POINTS**
> - In treating incontinence, it is important to determine the degree and cause of the problem. The patient's level of activity is also a factor in tailoring his treatment for incontinence.
> - Treatment options:
>   - anticholinergic drugs
>   - pelvic floor rehabilitation through stimulation and biofeedback
>   - injection of bulking material around the bladder neck to increase resistance
>   - artificial urinary sphincter
>   - gracilis myoplasty

The artificial urinary sphincter is usually deactivated after implantation for a period of 4 to 6 weeks to reduce local pressure on the urethra and to allow proper healing. The patient is warned that he will experience urinary incontinence during that time. Activation before healing is complete can result in pressure atrophy and cuff erosion through the urethra and hence failure of the procedure.

After activation, continence rate improves with time, and 90% of patients with this device have full continence by 1 year after implantation.[20] The most important complications associated with the device are infection and erosion. In one study the incidence of erosion reached 9%;[21] the risk of erosion increased with improper urethral manipulation (catheters) and previous exposure to pelvic radiation.

Gracilis myoplasty

Manipulation of the gracilis muscle, with its intact neurovascular bundle, has been used to improve urinary incontinence. The muscle is wrapped around the bulbar urethra in a fashion similar to that for the cuff of the artificial urinary sphincter. In a preliminary study Chancellor and colleagues[22] obtained encouraging results in a limited number of patients. This approach is an appropriate alternative to the artificial sphincter in patients with a high risk of complications, particularly after radiotherapy and cryotherapy.

This procedure is available only in special circumstances, for example, if the pelvic area has been irradiated or after failure of the artificial sphincter because of cuff erosion.

Conclusion

The patient described at the beginning of the article should expect some degree of urinary incontinence after the radical prostatectomy. The incontinence should gradually improve with time and pelvic-floor exercises. If the incontinence persists after 6 months, the patient should consult a urologist for a complete evaluation of the problem.

Erectile dysfunction*

In discussions of the consequences of radical prostatic surgery, and indeed most treatments for prostate cancer, the issue of "impotence" is always relevant.[23] However, the term "impotence" is often considered inappropriate, because it suggests global incompetence and may be perceived as unfair and inaccurate. Since the National Institutes of Health consensus conference on impotence in 1992,[24] the term "erectile dysfunction" has been preferred. The advantages of this medical term are that it encompasses different degrees of dysfunction and places the issue in a medical context, somewhat removed from common speech.

Defining erectile dysfunction

Erectile dysfunction is the persistent inability to attain and maintain penile erection sufficient for intercourse. It should be distinguished from sexual dysfunction, a broader term that would include a partner's physical problems, problems with intimacy or desire, and other less anatomically focused problems. Erectile dysfunction is confined to problems with rigidity of the penis and the assumption that these will interfere with normal sexual intercourse or activity.

It should be remembered that men can have orgasms independent of erection. Although the sensations of orgasm may arise from motor activity in sexual structures around the prostate, much of the impact of orgasm occurs in the brain. The word "climax" may capture the concept better than "orgasm," and recognizing these 2 components — the physical and the mental — may help in understanding why neither an erection nor a prostate gland is needed for orgasm. Thus, many men relate sensations of climax, even physical ones, after radical prostatectomy.[25]

It is also important to remember that erectile dysfunction is not a single

---

*This section by Dr. Jeremy P.W. Heaton.

condition; rather it occurs as a consequence of a variety of diseases and conditions affecting penile function. Normal erectile function depends on the near-perfect functioning of a highly vulnerable collection of blood vessels, nerves and fibrous tissue. Most men with erectile dysfunction have several problems that together cause a fault in the mechanics of erection.[26] From the time a man reaches maturity, the coordination of these mainly vascular phenomena begins to diminish, along with the ability to have an erection. For many years, the loss of potential may go unnoticed, but every man eventually realizes that his sexual response is not as robust, immediate or persistent as it used to be. Many men never lose entirely the ability to have an erection, but even so, they adapt their expectations to changing capabilities.

Each year, millions of North American men experience loss of erectile function. Their ability to have an erection reaches a point of delicate balance, where the slightest problem costs them an opportunity for intercourse, if not intimacy. Each year in Canada, more than 100 000 men enter a stage of their lives in which erection is unpredictable (estimated from the Massachusetts Male Aging Study[26]). This figure vastly exceeds the number of men undergoing surgery of the prostate area.

The physiology of erections

To understand the issues related to erectile dysfunction, it is necessary to appreciate how a sexual erection occurs. The brain receives a complex set of stimuli (some primitive, such as smell, others sophisticated, such as erotic images) and passes them through a specialized area in the midbrain that determines whether the erectile mechanism should be activated.[27] If so, a message is transmitted from the midbrain through the spinal cord. There, further signal processing occurs, and the message is dispersed into a multitude of nerve branches to cause tightening of the pelvic muscles and dilatation of the pelvic arteries. This dilatation allows blood to fill the spaces in the spongy tissue of the penis. If the blood pressure is high enough and the arteries allow enough blood into the penis, the core tissue (corpora cavernosa) swells and becomes tight against the tough fibrous outer casing (tunica albuginea). The filled corpora cavernosa become rigid and the penis becomes erect. The whole system, from brain to penile blood vessels, is held in a state of nonerection until the proper moment.

Causes of erectile dysfunction

The prostate is positioned astride the nerves and blood vessels that govern and effect erection. There are a multitude of nerves of various sizes, many grouped in bundles, each carrying some component of the erection message.

> **KEY POINTS**
> - Erectile dysfunction is the persistent inability to attain or maintain penile erection sufficient for intercourse.
> - Erectile dysfunction can result from normal loss of coordination of internal functions with age, but smoking speeds up the process, and diseases such as diabetes can also be a factor.
> - Stress, anxiety and worry also have an impact.

The muscles of the pelvis, which help in subtle ways to enhance erections, also support the prostate. Spontaneous erection cannot occur if too many of these structures are physically damaged. Thus, diseases that affect the nerves may have serious consequences for erectile function, as may conditions affecting the blood vessels. For example, diabetes, through damage to both nerves and arteries, is associated with early development of erectile dysfunction.[26] In addition, as men age, arterial elasticity is lost, and erectile capacity diminishes. Smoking is clearly associated with premature occurrence of erectile dysfunction.[26]

Beyond these potential causes of erectile dysfunction, the treatment of prostate cancer may interfere with erectile function. In fact, given the other factors just outlined, prostatic surgery may be the final step in reducing penile response below the threshold required for normal function. Even so-called "nerve-sparing" surgery can result in nerve and artery damage in this area.[28] All of the structures involved in erection — nerves, blood vessels and muscles — are susceptible to damage during prostate surgery or, indeed, any treatment of the prostate involving heat, cold or radiation.

Medical methods of treating prostate cancer can also interfere with the mechanisms of erection. For example, anti-androgen treatment required in the later stages of the disease[29] blocks the male sexual response at the same time as it blocks growth and reproduction of the cancer cells.

Stress, anxiety and worry — often experienced by men with prostate cancer — have an impact on erectile function, because they block excitation in the brain and relaxation of the blood vessels. Depression, another problem frequently experienced by people with cancer, as well as some other diseases of the brain (and even some character traits), may interfere with the brain chemistry necessary for initiating erection.

Preventive measures

In erectile dysfunction as in many other situations, the best treatment is prevention. Walsh and Donker[30] provided urologists with an understanding of the relevant anatomic structures that has allowed a sophisticated approach to surgical treatment of the disease: nerve-sparing radical prostatectomy. The intention in the nerve-sparing procedure is to avoid damaging the nerves behind the prostate by dissecting as close to the surface of the prostate as possible. Although in theory this might mean that cancer tissue at the surface of the prostate could be left behind, that risk is lower now that there is a much better understanding of who should undergo prostate surgery.[1]

Despite the introduction of a surgical procedure that conserves the nerves, a majority of men who undergo radical prostatectomy can still expect some degree of erectile dysfunction.[31] The early studies of nerve-sparing prostatectomy suggested that 84% of patients might remain potent,[32] 98% would retain some function and 52% would retain the ability to achieve vaginal penetration.[33] Subsequent series modified these expectations (suggesting that 75% might remain potent)[34] and stratified them for the effects of single or double nerve section — the results were better when only one nerve was cut.[35] The published rates of erectile dysfunction after nerve-sparing surgery have continued to rise, but the methods of examining patients before and after surgery, as reported in the erectile dysfunction literature, have not met the usual standards. A recent study[36] pointed out that of 11 patients who reported potency only 2 were satisfied with their sex life, yet 8 of 11 had nocturnal erections. These data demonstrated that it is difficult to ask precise questions and that there is much more to clinically relevant postoperative sexual function than mere penile response. Other studies have reported the rates of potency as 13.3%[31] and 41%[28] among patients with unilateral nerve preservation, and 31.9%[31] and 63%[28] among those with bilateral preservation; full erection has been reported for 9% of patients and partial erection for 38%.[37] There will be more studies with better data as the sophistication of measuring erectile dysfunction increases and the surgical techniques improve, such as with the use of nerve-finding devices and protocols.[38]

Other issues contributing to the successful preservation of potency have become better recognized. Age is a major factor in the societal prevalence of erectile dysfunction,[26] and it is not surprising that age has a significant impact on the incidence of erectile dysfunction after radical prostatectomy.[38] Nerve-sparing radical prostatectomy may influence arterial inflow, although the search for accessory vessels, an unexpected arterial supply within the surgical field, does not seem justified.[39] Surgery may have an effect that appears as veno-occlusive dysfunction on pharmacological testing, but this may also be seen if there is inadequate nerve supply and smooth-muscle deterioration; there is no reasonable causal relation that can be proposed for acute veno-occlusive dysfunction.

There are other consequences of surgery that affect sexual rehabilitation. For example, the penis becomes smaller,[40] and orgasm is altered.[25] Both the cancer and its treatment have a profound effect on the patient's psychological outlook, which will affect sexual function.[41] It should be noted that there are alternatives to surgery, which should be

> **KEY POINTS**
> - Every man undergoing radical prostate surgery should have some awareness not only that erectile function is at risk, but also that many treatment options are available.
> - Current treatments include intracavernous injection of prostaglandin, transurethral suppositories, drugs and various mechanical devices.

considered in terms of both sexual consequences and treatment efficacy.[23,42]

Treatment options

Patients with erectile dysfunction after prostatectomy have an advantage over men with spontaneous erectile dysfunction, because they know the reason for the problem. It is often easier to accept a side effect of needed treatment than to admit that the body is simply failing. Of the men who volunteer to discuss their erectile dysfunction with other patients or even with the media, more have a background of surgery than any other cause.

A man or a couple may consider treatment for surgically caused erectile dysfunction at any time after the diagnosis of prostate cancer. When surgery is presented as a treatment option, the patient must be told of the associated risks, but he can also be informed of the solutions for erectile dysfunction. Whether, how and when to treat the condition is a personal choice, but the patient needs information and advice to make such choices. Some urologists prefer to treat erectile dysfunction early — before or immediately after the urinary catheter is removed after surgery. The logic is that the earlier the arteries are "exercised," the better the prospects.[43] In addition, solving at least some of the problems associated with prostate cancer allows the physician and the patient to more effectively manage the intense disruption that cancer causes in a man's life and his relationships. Although there is as yet no perfect solution, research is continuing in this area.

Physicians should remind their patients that it will be months after surgery before healing restores optimal function. Nerve regrowth or repair may be slow and usually continues for 6 to 12 months after surgery.

A few years ago the only solution for erectile dysfunction after radical prostate surgery was the implantation of a penile prosthesis; some surgeons even started the process at the time of the initial procedure. Prosthetic devices are still an option for men unable to find another satisfactory solution. Vacuum erection devices, although effective and helpful for some, can be intrusive to the love-making cycle, may be uncomfortable, and may produce a cold penis (which may be uncomfortable for the partner).[44]

A major advance has been the advent of intracavernous injection of prostaglandin E_1 (alprostadil) (Caverject; Pharmacia & Upjohn, Mississauga, Ont.) (Table 1). Bypassing the mechanisms that may be damaged by aging, disease or surgery, prostaglandin — an agent that causes smooth-muscle relaxation by the cAMP pathway — can be delivered directly to the cavernosa (by injection), which results in penile erection in most men.[45] The drug is safe and has been well tested, the method of injection is much easier to learn than it first appears, and the rewards are clear — the opportunity to return to spontaneous intercourse and to reclaim that part of the patient's relationship and his self-esteem. The resulting erections are normal, and intercourse is not dangerous for either partner.

Prostaglandin can also be given in pellet form, delivered as a suppository to the urethra (MUSE; Vivus, Menlo Park, Calif.). This formulation is already in use in the United States and has recently become available in Canada (MUSE; Janssen Ortho, Toronto). Recent data indicate that it works after radical prostatectomy in about 40% of patients.[46]

There has been enormous interest in sildenafil (Viagra; Pfizer, New York), which received approval for treatment of erectile dysfunction in March 1998 in the US and March 1999 in Canada. This phosphodiesterase inhibitor, which comes in pill form and acts on smooth muscle by enhancing cyclic guanylyl monophosphate (cGMP) to facilitate erection, is effective in 43% of patients who have undergone treatment for prostate cancer.[47] Sildenafil increases cGMP only in cells that are activated, so the instructions for the patient are important. Sildenafil must be taken in prosexual circumstances, that is, sexual activity is needed for optimal effect. The most likely site of surgical damage causing erectile dysfunction is the nervi erigentes where they pass over the surface of the prostate. These nerves are essential for the proper activation of penile smooth-muscle second-messenger (cGMP) systems. This is one clear factor explaining the lower efficacy of sildenafil in men who have undergone radical prostatectomy relative to a cross-section of impotent men, in whom efficacy of up to 70%

Table 1: Options for treating erectile dysfunction after radical prostatectomy

Option	Benefit	Problems
Do nothing	Little "fuss"	May go against patient's, partner's and society's expectations
Intracavernous injection of prostaglandin	Prompt, reliable erection; probably most effective option	Intrusive
Transurethral suppository (prostaglandin)	Prompt and safe; 40% efficacy	Mildly intrusive
Older oral agents (e.g., yohimbine or trazodone)	Non-intrusive	Seldom effective
New oral agent (sildenafil)	Non-intrusive; efficacy probably similar to injection	Contraindicated if patient is receiving nitrates* 1-h onset time
Other new agents (e.g., phentolamine or apomorphine)	Non-intrusive; variable efficacy	Depends on drug class
Vacuum erection device	Effective	Intrusive, results in cold penis
Penile prosthesis	Effective	Invasive, irreversible

*It is unusual for patients who have undergone prostatectomy to use nitrates.

> **KEY POINTS**
> - A major advance for patients who have undergone prostate surgery has been the advent of intracavernous injection with prostaglandin, an artery-relaxing drug.
> - Sildenafil (Viagra), a drug that acts on the blood vessels to facilitate erection, is effective in many patients who have been treated for prostate cancer.
> - Other drugs in pill form are still undergoing clinical trials.

may be seen.[48,49] Full data from further trials will be welcome to better define the expected rate of success for sildenafil after radical prostatectomy. It can be expected that the success will vary with prior erectile status, age and the number of nerves preserved (none, one or both).

The principle of trying therapies that are known to be safe, that are not contraindicated and that may be effective is valid in all patients who have undergone radical prostatectomy. As in other patients with erectile dysfunction, sildenafil should be prescribed, according to the manufacturer's dosing recommendations, by knowledgeable physicians who understand the side-effect profile and the potential drug–drug interactions. The clear and absolute contraindication of any nitrate-containing medications has been well publicized. Minor and infrequent side effects include headaches, dyspepsia and flushing. The enthusiasm with which the popular press has reported the adoption of this drug and its social and adverse effects should be taken into account in managing patients, along with a critical appraisal of appropriate clinical information, of which there will be much more in the coming months and years.

Other medical alternatives include sublingual apomorphine (TAP Holdings, Deerfield, Ill.) and phentolamine taken by mouth (Vasomax; Zonagen/Schering Plough, Madison, NJ), either of which may be appropriate for erectile dysfunction related to prostate cancer. These compounds are still undergoing clinical trials and are not expected to receive approval until sometime in 1999 or 2000.

Other sources of prostaglandin E_1 are being developed, mainly for topical application. A combination injectable drug, consisting of a vasoactive intestinal polypeptide and phentolamine (Invicorp; Senetek, London, UK), is undergoing international trials, and new phosphodiesterase inhibitors that will work in a manner similar to sildenafil are being developed.

There may be benefit from early intracavernosal injection of prostaglandin after nerve-sparing radical prostatectomy. Montorsi and associates[43] found that 67% of patients given prostaglandin E_1 by this method early after their surgery had a satisfactory resumption of sexual function, compared with only 20% of those treated late. This is thought to be due to the antifibrotic properties of prostaglandin E_1. Other effective agents for erectile dysfunction may also have beneficial effects if started early after potentially "erectolytic" surgical injury.

For patients in whom oral and local prostaglandin therapy has failed, we use "triple therapy" by intracavernosal injection. This combination of prostaglandin E_1, phentolamine and papaverine was used before commercial preparations of prostaglandin E_1 became available and may be tried before the physician resorts to mechanical or surgical means of restoring rigidity.

Will conventional therapies for erectile dysfunction work after nerve-sparing radical prostatectomy? Given that there is no proven basis for selecting a particular therapy, treatment should be governed by the principles of goal-directed therapy[50] — whatever is safe and effective and suits the patient and his needs is reasonable.

The range of possible therapies is growing rapidly, which is fortunate given that most are satisfactory in fewer than 50% of patients after radical prostatectomy. In treating erectile dysfunction caused by prostatectomy, physicians will need good knowledge of the alternatives and an interest in trying different options. "Salvage therapy" includes a combination of drug therapy and penile prostheses.

Men who underwent prostatectomy many years ago may also want to consider treatment of any erectile problems that have resulted. However, the more severe the problem, the less likely that full erectile function will be recovered. In more difficult cases, more invasive solutions may be needed, although these may not be acceptable to all patients. In short, every man should have the choice of pursuing a remedy to his liking, but no one is guaranteed a satisfactory solution.

Conclusion

Erectile dysfunction occurring after treatment for prostate cancer brings with it yet another decision for the patient: the choice of whether to do anything about it. Even patients who do not have exceptional expectations of their family life should feel at liberty to ask questions about the problem. Physicians are now better informed about the issue than they were even 5 years ago, because of new interest in erectile dysfunction and vast improvements in managing the condition. The 68-year-old patient described at the beginning of this article has a better choice of treatment options and can expect more improvements in the future. In the whole complex of cancer care, erectile dysfunction is one area where the wishes and opinions of the patient must be considered first, and, finally, it is a problem that can be managed effectively in most men.

References

1. Goldenberg SL, Ramsey EW, Jewett MAS. Prostate cancer: 6. Surgical treatment of

localized disease. *CMAJ* 1998;159(10):1265-71. [Chapter 6 in this book.]
2. Warde P, Catton C, Gospodarowicz MK. Prostate cancer: 7. Radiation therapy for localized disease. *CMAJ* 1998;159(11):1381-8. [Chapter 7 in this book.]
3. Talcott JA, Rieker P, Propert HK, Clark JA, Winshnow KI, Loughlin KR, et al. Patient-reported incontinence after nerve-sparing radical prostatectomy. *J Natl Cancer Inst* 1997;89:1117-23.
4. Poore RE, McCullough DL, Jarow JP. Puboprostatic ligament sparing improves urinary continence after radical retropubic prostatectomy. *Urology* 1998;51:67-72.
5. Shelfo SW, Obeck C, Soloway MS. Update on bladder neck preservation during radical retropubic prostatectomy: impact on pathology outcome, anastomotic strictures and continence. *Urology* 1998;51:73-8.
6. Strassser H, Klima G, Poisel S, Horninger W, Bartsch G. Anatomy and innervation of the rhabdosphincter of the male urethra. *Prostate* 1996;28:24-31.
7. Strasser H, Frauscher F, Helweg G, Colleselli K, Reissigl A, Bartsch G. Transurethral ultrasound: evaluation of the anatomy and function of the rhabdosphincter of the male urethra. *J Urol* 1998;159:100-4.
8. Narayan P, Konety B, Aslam K, Aboseif S, Blumenfeld W, Tanagho E. Neuroanatomy of the external urethral sphincter: implications for urinary continence preservation during radical prostate surgery. *J Urol* 1995;153:337-41.
9. Milam DF, Franf JJ. Prevention and treatment of incontinence after radical prostatectomy. *Semin Urol Oncol* 1995;13:224-37.
10. Weldon VE, Tavel FR, Neuwirth H. Continence, potency and morbidity after radical perineal prostatectomy. *J Urol* 1997;158:1470-5.
11. Kaye KW, Creed KE, Wilson GJ, D'Antuono M, Dawkins HJ. Urinary incontinence after radical retropubic prostatectomy. Analysis and synthesis of contributing factors: a unified concept. *Br J Urol* 1997;80:444-501.
12. Donnellan SM, Duncan HJ, MacGregor RJ, Russell JM. Prospective assessment of incontinence after radical retropubic prostatectomy: objective and subjective analysis. *Urology* 1997;49:225-30.
13. Hammerer P, Huland H. Urodynamic evaluation of changes in urinary control after radical retropubic prostatectomy. *J Urol* 1997;157:233-6.
14. Desautel MG, Kapoor R, Badlani GH. Sphincteric incontinence: the primary cause of post-prostatectomy incontinence in patients with prostate cancer. *Neurourol Urodyn* 1997;16:153-60.
15. Minervini R, Felipetto R, Morelli G, Fontana N, Fiorentini L. Urodynamic evaluation of urinary incontinence following radical prostatectomy: our experience. *Acta Urol Belg* 1996;64:5-8.
16. Goluboff ET, Chang DT, Olsson CA, Kaplan SA. Urodynamics and the etiology of post-prostatectomy urinary incontinence: the initial Columbia experience. *J Urol* 1995;153:1034-7.
17. Harris JL. Treatment of post-prostatectomy urinary incontinence with behavioral methods. *Clin Nurse Spec* 1997;11:159-63.
18. Waintein MA, Klutke CG. Antegrade technique of collagen injection for postprostatectomy stress incontinence: the Washington University experience. *World J Urol* 1997;15:310-5.
19. Rosen M. A simple artificial implantable sphincter. *Br J Urol* 1976;48:675-80.

20. Fleshner N, Herschorn S. The artificial urinary sphincter for post-radical prostatectomy incontinence: impact on urinary symptoms and quality of life. *J Urol* 1996;155:1260-4.
21. Martins FE, Boyd SD. Post-operative risk factors associated with urinary sphincter infection-erosion. *Br J Urol* 1995;75:354-8.
22. Chancellor MB, Watanabe T, Rivas DA, Hong RD, Kumon H, Ozawa H, et al. Gracilis urethral myoplasty: preliminary experience using an autologous urinary sphincter for post-prostatectomy incontinence. *J Urol* 1997;158:1372-5.
23. Robinson JW, Dufour MS, Fung TS. Erectile functioning of men treated for prostate carcinoma. *Cancer* 1997;79:538-44.
24. NIH Consensus Development Panel on Impotence. Impotence [NIH consensus conference]. *JAMA* 1993;270:83-90.
25. Koeman M, van Driel MF, Schultz WC, Mensink HJ. Orgasm after radical prostatectomy. *Br J Urol* 1996;77:861-4.
26. Feldman HA, Goldstein I, Hatzichristou DG, Krane RJ, McKinlay JB. Impotence and its medical and psychosocial correlates: results of the Massachusetts Male Aging Study. *J Urol* 1994;151:54-61.
27. Giuliano FA, Rampin O, Benoit G, Jardin A. Neural control of penile erection. *Urol Clin North Am* 1995;22:747-66.
28. Catalona WJ, Basler JW. Return of erections and urinary continence following nerve sparing radical retropubic prostatectomy. *J Urol* 1993;150:905-7.
29. Gleave ME, Bruchovsky N, Moore MJ, Venner P. Prostate cancer: 9. Treatment of advanced disease. *CMAJ* 1999;160(2):225-32. [Chapter 9 in this book.]
30. Walsh PC, Donker PJ. Impotence following radical prostatectomy: insight into etiology and prevention. *J Urol* 1982;128:492-7.
31. Geary ES, Dendinger TE, Freiha FS, Stamey TA. Nerve sparing radical prostatectomy: a different view. *J Urol* 1995;154:145-9.
32. Eggleston JC, Walsh PC. Radical prostatectomy with preservation of sexual function: pathological findings in the first 100 cases. *J Urol* 1985;134(6):1146-8.
33. Catalona WJ, Dresner SM. Nerve-sparing radical prostatectomy: extraprostatic tumor extension and preservation of erectile function. *J Urol* 1985;134(6):1149-51.
34. Walsh PC, Schlegel PN. Radical pelvic surgery with preservation of sexual function. *Ann Surg* 1988;208(4):391-400.
35. Quinlan DM, Epstein JI, Carter BS, Walsh PC. Sexual function following radical prostatectomy: influence of preservation of neurovascular bundles. *J Urol* 1991;145(5):998-1002.
36. Lerner SE, Richards SL, Benet AE, Kahan NZ, Fleischmann JD, Melman A. [Detailed evaluation of sexual function after radical prostatectomy: Is patient satisfaction correlated with the quality of erections?] *Prog Urol* 1996;6(4):552-7.
37. Jonler M, Messing EM, Rhodes PR, Bruskewitz RC. Sequelae of radical prostatectomy. *Br J Urol* 1994;74(3):352-8.
38. Klotz L, Herschorn S. Early experience with intraoperative cavernous nerve stimulation during nerve-sparing radical prostatectomy. *Urology* 1998;52:537-42.
39. Polascik TJ, Walsh PC. Radical retropubic prostatectomy: the influence of accessory pudendal arteries on the recovery of sexual function. *J Urol* 1995;154(1):150-2.
40. McCullough AR, Lepor H. The loss of penile length and circumference in impotent

men after nerve sparing radical prostatectomy. *J Urol* 1988;159(5):S98.
41. Schover LR. Sexual rehabilitation after treatment for prostate cancer. *Cancer* 1993;71(3 Suppl):1024-30.
42. Mantz CA, Song P, Farhangi E, Nautiyal J, Awan A, Ignacio L, et al. Potency probability following conformal megavoltage radiotherapy using conventional doses for localized prostate cancer. *Int J Radiat Oncol Biol Phys* 1997;37(3):551-7.
43. Montorsi F, Guazzoni G, Strambi LF, Da Pozzo LF, Nava L, Barbieri L, et al. Recovery of spontaneous erectile function after nerve-sparing radical retropubic prostatectomy with and without early intracavernous injections of alprostadil: results of a prospective, randomized trial. *J Urol* 1997;158:1408-10.
44. Opsomer RJ, Wese FX, De Groote P, Van Cangh PJ. The external vacuum device in the management of erectile dysfunction. *Acta Urol Belg* 1997;65(4):13-6.
45. Soderdahl DW, Thrasher JB, Hansberry KL. Intracavernosal drug-induced erection therapy versus external vacuum devices in the treatment of erectile dysfunction. *Br J Urol* 1997;79:952-7.
46. Costabile RA, Spevak M, Fishman IJ, Govier FE, Hellstrom WJG, Shabsigh R, et al. Efficacy and safety of transurethral alprostadil in patients with erectile dysfunction following radical prostatectomy. *J Urol* 1998;160:1325-8.
47. Zippe CD, Kedia AW, Kedia K, Nelson DR, Agarwal A. Treatment of erectile dysfunction after radical prostatectomy with sildenafil citrate (Viagra). *Urology* 1998;52(6):963-6.
48. Goldstein I, Lue TF, Padma-Nathan H, Rosen RC, Steers WD, Wicker P. Oral sildenafil in the treatment of erectile dysfunction. Sildenafil Study Group. [Published erratum appears in *N Engl J Med* 1998;339(1):59.] *N Engl J Med* 1998;338(20):1397-404.
49. Montorsi F, McDermott TE, Morgan R, Olsson A, Schultz A, Kirkeby HJ, et al. Efficacy and safety of fixed-dose oral sildenafil in the treatment of erectile dysfunction of various etiologies. *Urology* 1999;53(5):1011-8.
50. Lue TF. Impotence: a patient's goal-directed approach to treatment. *World J Urol* 1990;8:67-74.

9

Treatment of advanced disease

Martin E. Gleave, MD; Nick Bruchovsky, MD, PhD;
Malcolm J. Moore, MD; Peter Venner, BMSc, MD

> A 70-year-old man is referred to a urologist for recommendations on the management of metastatic prostate cancer. His cancer was diagnosed 5 years ago, and he underwent radical prostatectomy at that time. The tumour was confined to the prostate gland (Gleason score 7), and during surgery the lymph nodes were assessed as being clear of cancer. Before the surgery, the patient's prostate-specific antigen (PSA) level had been 8 ng/mL. After the prostatectomy, PSA was at first undetectable, but recently the PSA level rose to 2 ng/mL and then, at the most recent test, to 16 ng/mL. A bone scan was ordered to investigate back discomfort, which has been persistent but easily controlled with acetaminophen. Unfortunately, the bone scan shows several sites of metastatic disease. The man's medical history includes type 2 diabetes, which has developed during the past 3 years and which is controlled by diet, as well as asymptomatic hypertension, which is managed by means of a thiazide diuretic. The patient asks what treatments are available, what impact they are likely to have on his disease and what risks are associated with the therapies.

The patient in this case exemplifies the consequences of failed local therapies and presents a scenario that is altogether too familiar to any practitioner who cares for men with prostate cancer. Current systemic therapies include alterations in the patient's hormonal milieu or the use of a cytotoxic agent. The impact of both approaches is discussed here.

Androgens and the prostate gland

The male sex hormones are collectively known as androgens — from the

Greek *andros* (man) and *gennan* (to produce). Testosterone is the principal circulating androgen in men, and its presence is necessary for normal development of the penis, scrotum, testicles and male secondary sex characteristics at puberty. Testicular androgens are critical in the formation of the prostate gland in the embryo and for its normal function throughout adulthood, including production of prostate-specific antigen (PSA).

Testosterone has long been implicated as a possible promoter of prostatic cancer growth. Prostate cancer does not develop in eunuchs or other men castrated before puberty, and latent prostate cancer is less frequent among men with cirrhosis, who often have low testosterone levels.

The normal pathways for endocrine control of gonadal function are summarized in Fig. 1. Testosterone synthesized in the testes is a precursor for 90% of the dihydrotestosterone produced in the prostate; the remaining 10% is derived from the less-potent adrenal androgens — androstenedione and dehydroepiandrosterone — and from extrinsic

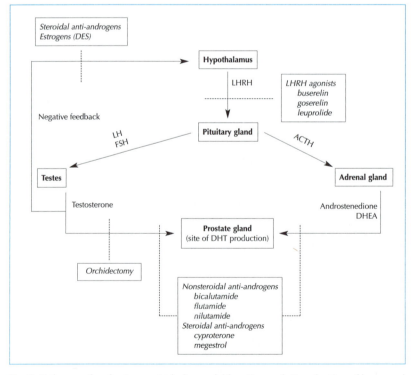

Fig. 1: Pathways of endocrine control of gonadal function and sites of action of hormonal agents. The tissues involved in regulation of gonadal function are indicated by bold type. Direction of action of endocrines is indicated by arrows. Dotted lines indicate where various hormonal agents (shown in italic) interfere with normal endocrine flow. ACTH = adrenocorticotropic hormone, DES = diethylstilbestrol, DHEA = dehydroepiandrosterone, DHT = dihydrotestosterone, FSH = follicle-stimulating hormone, LH = luteinizing hormone, LHRH = luteinizing hormone-releasing hormone.

sources. Testosterone provides a negative feedback signal for the hypothalamic secretion of luteinizing hormone-releasing hormone (LHRH) and, subsequently, release of luteinizing hormone from the pituitary gland.

Testosterone circulates in association with 2 major plasma proteins: sex-hormone-binding globulin and albumin. Only 2% of the testosterone is unbound and available for diffusion into the target cell, where it is converted to dihydrotestosterone by the enzyme 5-α-reductase.[1] Dihydrotestosterone then binds to and activates androgen receptors, which bind to the promoter regions of specific genes, thereby regulating transcription and hence protein synthesis, cell growth and differentiation.[2]

> **KEY POINTS**
> - Suppression of testosterone (androgen ablation) is effective in checking the growth of prostate cancer and reducing tumour volume, although this treatment will not eliminate all malignant cells.
> - Androgen withdrawal produces a response in up to 80% of patients with advanced prostate cancer; the median progression-free survival is 2–3 years.

No treatment equals or surpasses androgen ablation in checking the growth of prostate cancer and reducing tumour volume; biochemical and objective responses are achieved in 80% of patients.[3-11] Withdrawal of androgen induces apoptosis, a form of programmed cell death, in normal and malignant prostatic epithelial cells. However, this fails to eliminate the entire population of malignant cells, and progression to androgen independence almost inevitably occurs, which leads to the development of symptoms (e.g., bone pain, weight loss and fatigue) and death.

Progression to androgen independence is a complex process. It involves selection and growth of pre-existing clones of androgen-independent cells; adaptive up-regulation (i.e., increased expression) of genes that help the cancer cells survive and grow after androgen ablation; and androgen-receptor mutations or interactions with alternative transcription factors.[12] Better understanding of the molecular basis of apoptosis and progression to androgen independence will provide clinicians with novel therapeutic targets in the future.

Androgen withdrawal therapy

The ablation of testicular function in the palliative treatment of prostate cancer was first attempted in the 1930s by means of radiation of the testes. This proved less effective than surgical removal, which was introduced a decade later.[3] Bilateral orchidectomy has become the gold standard of hormonal therapy for metastatic prostate cancer. Its advantages include low cost, low morbidity and the avoidance of compliance problems that may arise with drug therapy. However, the psychologic trauma associated with surgical castration has increased the use of medical castration.

Over the past 2 decades, drugs affecting the hypothalamic production of LHRH and those blocking the peripheral effects of androgens (steroidal and nonsteroidal anti-androgens) have been used alone and in various combinations to achieve medical castration. The advent of these agents has increased the options for suppressing the influence of androgens on the growth of prostate cancer (Table 1). The general side effects of androgen ablation include hot flushes, gynecomastia, loss of libido and potency, lethargy, and loss of bone and muscle mass over time.

Several classes of drugs induce castrate levels of testosterone by suppressing the release of luteinizing hormone from the pituitary gland. For example, diethylstilbestrol (DES) suppresses hypothalamic release of LHRH and increases levels of testosterone-binding globulin; these effects combine to decrease the serum level of free testosterone. DES is the least expensive of the synthetic estrogens, and castrate testosterone levels are achieved at doses of 1 mg/day.[4] However, its low cost must be weighed against the increased risk of thromboembolic and cardiovascular complications.[4]

LHRH agonists include goserelin and leuprolide (available as monthly subcutaneous and intramuscular injections respectively and, more recently, as 3-month formulations) and buserelin (available as a 2-month depot formulation). Pulsatile release of LHRH from the hypothalamus normally stimulates the release of luteinizing hormone from the pituitary gland, but when this periodicity is disrupted by continuous administration of LHRH agonists, hypothalamic regulation of the pituitary is lost.

Table 1: Relative benefits of various forms of medical castration*

Benefit	Therapeutic option; degree of benefit					
	LHRH agonist alone	CPA alone	Lead-in CPA + CAB†	CAB + nonsteroidal anti-androgen	CAB + CPA	CPA + DES
Rapid onset	–	+	++	+	+	++
Reversibility	++	++	++	++	++	++
Absence of flare	–	++	++	+	+	++
Absence of hot flushes	–	+	+	–	+	+
Low toxicity	+	+	++	–	+	+
Low cost	–	+	–	–	–	++
Ease of administration	++	++	+	+	+	++

Note: LHRH = luteinizing hormone-releasing hormone, CPA = cyproterone acetate, CAB = combined androgen blockade (LHRH agonist + steroidal anti-androgen), DES = diethylstilbestrol.
*The relative merits assigned in this table represent the authors' views, which are based on the use of multiple drug regimens over the years to produce androgen ablation.
†CPA used as lead-in therapy for first month to prevent flare.

LHRH agonists produce a biphasic response — an initial rise in levels of luteinizing hormone and testosterone, termed the "flare phenomenon," followed in 2 weeks by a fall in these levels.[5] The flare phenomenon can be prevented by administering cyproterone acetate or DES 1 week before the LHRH agonist; alternatively, it can be blocked by nonsteroidal anti-androgens.[6] Although LHRH agonists appear equivalent to DES and orchidectomy, the flare phenomenon is one disadvantage of using these drugs alone. Their main advantages are reversibility and the avoidance of cardiovascular complications, but these are achieved at high cost ($400/month).

Anti-androgens compete with androgens for receptor sites in target cells. Current indications for their use are outlined in Table 2. The nonsteroidal anti-androgens — which include bicalutamide, flutamide and nilutamide — have no direct gonadotropic or progestational effects and therefore do not suppress testosterone levels. Most studies do not support the use of nonsteroidal anti-androgens alone,[6] although recent data suggest that higher-dose (150 mg/day) bicalutamide monotherapy may be equivalent to surgical castration.[7] The reported side effects of these nonsteroidal anti-androgens are summarized in Table 3.

Steroidal anti-androgens (cyproterone acetate and megestrol) have progestational activity in addition to their anti-androgenic activity at peripheral receptors; thus, they inhibit secretion of gonadotropin and production of testosterone.[6] The combination of low-dose cyproterone acetate (50 mg twice daily) and mini-dose DES (0.1 mg daily) achieves potent androgen ablation at one-third the cost of LHRH agonists.[9] The advantages of steroidal anti-androgens include reversibility, suppression of hot flushes and

Table 2: Indications for use of anti-androgens

To prevent the flare phenomenon during the first month of LHRH agonist treatment:
  cyproterone acetate (50 mg twice daily) plus DES (0.1 mg daily)
  or cyproterone acetate (150 mg orally, twice daily)
  or a nonsteroidal anti-androgen

To treat hot flushes after medical or surgical castration:
  cyproterone acetate (50 mg once daily)

To treat biochemical (indicated by rising PSA level) or clinical progression of disease in patients treated with LHRH agonists, orchidectomy or low-dose cyproterone acetate and mini-dose DES: 3-month trial with a nonsteroidal anti-androgen (bicalutamide, flutamide or nilutamide), to be continued only if there is a decrease in serum PSA level

Note: PSA = prostate-specific antigen.

Table 3: Summary of side effects of nonsteroidal anti-androgens

Anti-androgen	Side effects
Bicalutamide[8]	Gynecomastia (25%)
Nilutamide[6]	Decreased adaptation of vision to darkness (33%)
	Nausea (25%)
	Alcohol intolerance (20%)
	Possibility of interstitial pneumonitis
Flutamide[9,11]	Gynecomastia (60%)
	Diarrhea (10%)
	Nausea
	Possibility of idiosyncratic hepatocellular toxicity resulting in death

intermediate expense. Specific side effects include the potential for fatigue and depression.[9]

Responses to androgen withdrawal therapy

Up to 80% of patients with metastatic disease exhibit objective responses to androgen ablation; median overall progression-free survival is 23 to 37 months.[8,10,11] Serum PSA level remains the most useful indication of response and prognosis in these patients. Almost all treated patients have an initial response accompanied by a rapid decrease in serum PSA, which falls into the normal range in about 70% of patients.

The level of serum PSA after 6 months of treatment indicates whether the response will be prolonged.[13–15] PSA levels greater than 4 ng/mL after 6 months of therapy are associated with a median survival of 18 months, whereas levels below 4 ng/mL are associated with a median survival of 40 months.[13–15] Furthermore, a rising PSA level is the earliest sign of progression, predating clinical recurrence by 6 to 12 months.

The flutamide withdrawal syndrome[6] is characterized by a 50% decrease in serum PSA level after discontinuation of this anti-androgen. Despite its name, the syndrome has been reported in approximately 20% of patients after discontinuation of both steroidal and nonsteroidal anti-androgens. This phenomenon highlights the potential role for androgen receptor mutations and anti-androgens in tumour progression and implies that partial antagonists (like nonsteroidal anti-androgens) may become partial agonists during progression to androgen independence, probably because of subtle changes in androgen receptor structure and protein–protein interactions.

Controversial issues in advanced prostate cancer

Is combined androgen blockade superior to castration alone?

The term "combined androgen blockade" describes the addition of an anti-androgen to medical or surgical castration to block the action of residual (adrenal) androgens. Although this concept dates back to 1945[16] and has been the subject of randomized controlled trials for 15 years, it remains controversial.

Dihydrotestosterone is detectable in prostate tissue after castration. Early attempts to eliminate the source of residual androgens by adrenalectomy were ineffective, but the development of nonsteroidal anti-androgens in the late 1970s revived interest in this approach. However, the numerous trials conducted to date have had mixed results. For example, a National Cancer Institute (NCI) intergroup study[10] found that among patients with previously untreated metastatic prostate cancer, duration of progression-free and median survival was statistically significantly longer for those treated with a combination of the LHRH agonist leuprolide and the nonsteroidal anti-androgen flutamide than for those treated with leuprolide and placebo. However, critics have correctly pointed out that leuprolide therapy may be subject to problems with compliance and that the inferior results for leuprolide with placebo may have resulted from untreated flare.

> **KEY POINTS**
> - The choice of androgen ablation therapy for advanced prostate cancer depends on the philosophy of the physician, patient preferences and cost.
> - Orchidectomy is still the most cost-effective therapy for metastatic prostate cancer.
> - Androgen withdrawal therapies, which are equivalent to orchidectomy, are reversible and offer flexibility and the possiblity of many new approaches.
> - The main obstacle to improving survival and quality of life in patients with advanced prostate cancer is progression to androgen independence, whereby tumour cells survive despite the absence of androgens.
> - Accumulating evidence supports the initiation of androgen ablation as soon as locally advanced, recurrent or metastatic disease is diagnosed.

The difficulty in analysing and integrating the results of numerous trials arises from heterogeneity in type of castration and type of anti-androgen, as well as differences in study design, randomization procedures, assessment of treatment outcomes, statistical evaluation and length of follow-up. A meta-analysis of 22 randomized trials evaluating combined androgen blockade found no significant improvement in 5-year survival.[11] Continuing debate regarding this therapy prompted the largest trial to date for advanced prostate cancer, in which 1387 patients were randomly chosen to undergo orchidectomy combined with either flutamide or placebo; recent reports indicate no differences in survival in any subgroup.[17]

One explanation for the differences between this study and the earlier NCI intergroup study is that untreated flare with LHRH monotherapy adversely affects overall survival. At present, the data do not convincingly show a benefit of combined androgen blockade over castration alone for patients with metastatic prostate cancer, which implies that the role for adrenal androgens in disease progression after castration is insignificant.

When should androgen ablation be initiated?

Although early studies found that delayed and immediate endocrine therapy were equivalent, any apparent benefit of immediate therapy may have been obscured by the cardiovascular side effects of DES.[18] Furthermore, theoretical and animal-model data suggest that early androgen ablation is more effective.[19] A recent randomized controlled study of patients with locally advanced disease compared radiation therapy plus 3 years of adjuvant hormone therapy with radiation therapy initially plus hormone therapy only at disease recurrence; 5-year overall survival was significantly better in the first group.[20] The results of a British study comparing early and delayed endocrine therapy in metastatic prostate cancer also supported immediate therapy.[21] Taken together, accumulating evidence supports initiation of treatment as soon as locally advanced, recurrent or metastatic disease is diagnosed.

Quality-of-life issues

Patients with metastatic prostate cancer have a median survival time of only 2–3 years, so there is not enough time for the long-term effects of androgen ablation to be manifested; therefore, these effects are not clinically relevant. However, awareness of potential adverse effects of long-term continuous androgen ablation is increasing. PSA testing has shifted diagnosis to an earlier stage, which means that diagnosis of locally advanced or metastatic disease is less frequent, and diagnosis of clinically confined disease (stage T1c or T2) more frequent. Moreover, PSA detection of recurrence after radical prostatectomy or radiotherapy identifies men who may benefit from early therapy and who may have a life expectancy exceeding 10 years. These trends are forcing clinicians to balance the potential benefits of early adjuvant therapy with the risks of metabolic complications and the increased expense associated with long-term continuous androgen withdrawal therapy. The metabolic complications include osteoporosis and fractures, loss of muscle mass, anemia, fatigue and lethargy, changes in lipid profile (with an increased risk of cardiovascular complications), glucose intolerance and personality changes, including depression or irritability.

New approaches that use reversible medical castration are being studied to reduce the negative impact of androgen ablation on quality of life, with the realization that androgen withdrawal therapy is rarely curative, that combined androgen blockade is not superior to orchidectomy and that progression to androgen independence is initiated and accelerated by androgen withdrawal. The treatment goal is no longer to kill all cancer cells by maximizing androgen ablation; rather, the goal is now to regain biological control of the growth of tumour cells, as well as their response to subsequent androgen ablation.

Intermittent androgen suppression is based on the hypothesis that if tumour cells that have survived androgen withdrawal are forced along a normal pathway of differentiation by re-exposure to androgen (i.e., interruption of the medical castration therapy), then apoptotic potential may be restored and progression to androgen independence delayed. Experimental animal data and clinical studies support this hypothesis.[22] Androgen withdrawal therapy was continued for 9 months, after which medications were discontinued (Fig. 2). When serum PSA levels increased to 10–20 ng/mL, treatment was resumed. The cycle of treatment followed by no treatment was repeated until regulation of PSA level became androgen-independent. Nearly half of each cycle involved no treatment, and off-treatment periods were associated with an improved sense of well-being and recovery of libido and potency in the men who reported sexual function before the start of therapy.

Observations from preliminary studies suggest that intermittent androgen suppression does not have a negative impact on time to progression or survival. This treatment option offers clinicians an opportunity to improve quality of life by balancing the benefits of immediate androgen ablation (i.e., delayed progression and prolonged survival) while reducing treatment-related side effects and expense. Phase III randomized studies of the efficacy of intermittent androgen suppression have been initiated in Canada, the United States and Europe. Until survival data are available, it should be considered an investigational form of therapy.

Another approach to reduce the side effects of therapy is the concept of sequential androgen blockade.[23] The relative potency of nonsteroidal anti-androgens such as flutamide is increased by inhibiting conversion of testosterone to the more potent dihydrotestosterone, which thereby obviates the necessity for castrate levels of testosterone. The usual side effects of androgen ablation are avoided because testosterone levels are not reduced. Libido and potency are preserved in most patients. Further follow-up and comparative studies are needed to determine whether time to progression or survival are adversely affected.

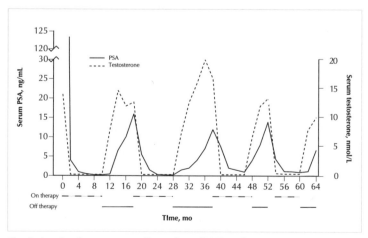

Fig. 2: Levels of prostate-specific antigen (PSA) and testosterone in serum of patients treated with intermittent androgen suppression.

Hormone-refractory prostate cancer

Hormone-refractory prostate cancer, defined as symptomatic prostate cancer that is progressing despite optimal hormone therapy, is disabling and incurable. Patients have a serum testosterone level in the castrate range and, typically, the serum level of PSA is rising. Hormone-refractory prostate cancer is associated with a symptom complex that includes progressive bone metastases that may be painful, fatigue, weight loss and, occasionally, bone marrow failure.

> **KEY POINTS**
> - Metastatic prostate cancer frequently progresses to a hormone-refractory stage that is disabling and incurable.
> - This stage is associated with progressive painful bony metastases, fatigue, weight loss and, occasionally, bone marrow failure.

At this stage of prostate cancer, radionuclide bone scans often reveal new progressive lesions, and diagnostic imaging procedures occasionally show soft-tissue lesions. Once symptoms develop, most patients become essentially incapacitated, and median survival time is 9–12 months.[24] These patients are generally elderly, they often have concurrent medical problems, and their bone marrow function may be compromised as a result of both disease and prior radiation therapy. They are generally intolerant of aggressive cytotoxic therapies.

With the widespread use of PSA testing, many patients receiving hormone therapy (but "resistant" to it) are now presenting when their PSA level first begins to rise, rather than when clinical symptoms develop. An apparent increase in median survival time, from 6–9 months in older studies of chemotherapy to 10–13 months in more recent ones, is probably due to initiation of treatment when PSA elevation indicates hormone-refractory disease, rather than when clinical progression becomes apparent.[24] As yet, no systemic therapies have been shown to have any meaningful impact on survival in randomized trials. Thus, any therapy must be recommended in light of its ability to diminish disease-related symptoms and improve quality of life.

Chemotherapy in hormone-refractory prostate cancer

Early studies of chemotherapy examined a variety of single agents and drug combinations.[25] Even though "responses" were noted (according to the criteria established by that group), they were infrequent; there was no impact on survival and, therefore, no convincing standard regimen was established. Many investigators concluded that, given the potential for toxic effects and the lack of demonstrable benefit, chemotherapy had little or no role in the management of hormone-refractory prostate cancer.[24]

More recently, many researchers have used changes in PSA level to infer that chemotherapy *is* effective in this form of the disease. However, some caution must be exercised in interpreting PSA changes in these patients. PSA is not as good an indicator of disease bulk in this situation as it is in earlier-stage disease. In addition, changes in PSA level do not provide information about the balance between toxic effects of the treatment and reduction of tumour-related symptoms. Furthermore, many agents reduce PSA gene expression without inducing death of tumour cells.

> **KEY POINTS**
> - Although testing for prostate-specific antigen is helping to identify hormone-refractory prostate cancer earlier, to date no therapies have had any meaningful effect on survival.
> - Any treatment must be recommended in light of its ability to reduce symptoms and improve quality of life.
> - The tremendous cost and overall burden that hormone-refractory prostate cancer places on patients and society has led to increased efforts to find new therapies and to re-examine some older regimens for their potential palliative benefit.

Recognition of the tremendous cost and overall burden that hormone-refractory prostate cancer places on patients and society has contributed to a continuing effort to develop and investigate new therapies. The most recent studies have investigated mitoxantrone plus prednisone, estramustine combinations and suramin. In addition, some older, well-tolerated regimens, such as cyclophosphamide given orally, are being re-examined for their potential palliative benefit.

Mitoxantrone plus prednisone

Mitoxantrone is an anthracenedione, a chemotherapy agent that acts by inhibiting topo-isomerase II. In initial studies of mitoxantrone in hormone-refractory prostate cancer the objective response rate was relatively low, but a larger number of patients experienced significant reduction of pain.[25] Recognizing that symptom control is important and that prolonging survival may not be a realistic outcome, pain relief may be regarded as a valid objective.

The primary endpoint in these trials was a "palliative response," defined as a significant reduction in pain with no increase in use of analgesics, or a 35% decrease in use of analgesics without any increase in pain.[26] On the basis of these criteria, a phase III study was undertaken to compare prednisone with prednisone plus mitoxantrone. A palliative response was achieved in 30 (38%) of 80 patients receiving the combined treatment and in only 17 (21%) of 81 who received prednisone alone ($p = 0.025$).[27] The median duration of the palliative response was longer for the combination treatment than for prednisone alone (43 and 18 weeks respectively; $p < 0.001$).

The patients who met the criteria for a palliative response also had improvements in most domains on quality-of-life scales, including highly significant improvements in overall well-being. There was no significant improvement in survival. A fall in PSA level of 75% or more was seen in 27% of those who received mitoxantrone plus prednisone and in only 9% of those who received prednisone alone. Mitoxantrone was well-tolerated, and the incidence of serious toxic effects was low. There was no evidence of deterioration in any quality-of-life domains associated with chemotherapy.

Estramustine combinations

Estramustine, composed of nornitrogen mustard and estradiol joined by a carbamate ester linkage, produces cytotoxic effects independent of its alkylating and hormonal constituents. The antineoplastic effects of estramustine are believed to arise from its effects on microtubule-associated proteins and consequent disruption of mitosis.

Estramustine has been extensively tested in patients with hormone-refractory prostate cancer, and as a single agent its benefits are minimal. However, it has been evaluated recently in combination with chemotherapeutic agents with which it has synergistic cytotoxicity in vitro (e.g., vinblastine, etoposide and paclitaxel). The results of 3 phase II trials of the combined regimen of estramustine and vinblastine have recently been published.[28]

The PSA response rate — defined as the percentage of patients with a decrease in PSA level of 50% or greater — for the 88 patients in the combined estramustine–vinblastine studies was 42%.[28] Partial responses were noted in 6 (24%) of 25 patients with bidimensionally measurable non-osseous disease. Recently completely randomized trials comparing estramustine plus vinblastine with vinblastine alone (by the Hoosier Oncology Group) and with estramustine alone (by EORTC, the European Organization for Research and Treatment of Cancer) will better define the role of estramustine in hormone-refractory prostate cancer.

Recent phase II studies evaluating estramustine plus etoposide and estramustine plus paclitaxel have also been reported.[29,30] Both showed activity similar to that reported for estramustine plus vinblastine; however, these single-study results are early, and the toxic effects of these regimens may be a problem.

Suramin

Suramin was originally synthesized 80 years ago and has been used to treat a variety of parasitic diseases. In the 1980s its cytotoxic activity against human prostatic cell lines in vitro was noted.[31] Although some clinical trials demonstrated activity against hormone-refractory prostate cancer, the relative merits of this agent are a subject of controversy. Eisenberger and colleagues[32] found a response in 6 of 12 patients with measurable disease, a reduction in PSA level of at least 50% in 77% of patients (24/31) and a reduction of 75% in 55% (17/31).

However, suramin is known to inhibit PSA release, and 9 of the 24 patients with a decrease in PSA level of 50% or more had evidence of disease progression at the same time. Treatment was discontinued in 80% of the patients (28/35) because of dose-limiting toxic effects, which presented primarily as a syndrome of fatigue, malaise and lethargy. Thus the palliative benefit of such a regimen must be questioned.

Suramin suppresses adrenocortical function and is given in conjunction with hydrocortisone. The concomitant use of steroids has made it difficult to establish the response attributable to suramin. In a study in which patients received suramin only, after progression on corticosteroids alone, only minimal activity was seen; there was no demonstrable response in patients with measurable disease.[33] A better understanding of suramin will come from a large, recently completed North American trial involving 500 patients, randomly chosen to receive suramin plus hydrocortisone or hydrocortisone alone.

Conclusion

Better therapies are needed for the prevention and treatment of hormone-refractory prostate cancer. Novel approaches currently being tested in early clinical trials include angiogenesis inhibitors, immunological therapies, gene therapy and differentiation therapies. Because of the high incidence of bone metastases in metastatic prostate cancer and their potential devastating effects, the role of bone-stabilizing agents, such as the bisphosphonates, is being explored in phase III studies.

However, until we have identified treatments that significantly affect survival, we must focus on relieving patients' distress and improving their overall quality of life. To this end, the only drug therapy with a documented benefit is the combination of mitoxantrone and prednisone. Although far from a cure, this combination has a role in treating symptomatic patients and can be the standard against which newer therapies are compared.

To return to the patient described at the beginning of this article, it seems that there is both good news and bad news for him. The bad news is that he cannot be cured and that available hormonal therapies produce side effects that will undoubtedly compromise his quality of life. The good news is that hormone therapies will almost certainly control his disease for a few years, and, if hormone-resistant disease develops, there is a chemotherapy regimen of known efficacy to palliate his symptoms.

Although of little immediate benefit to this patient, the randomized controlled trial of intermittent hormone therapy may change the way we care for patients in the future. Furthermore, we now have a chemotherapy standard and a method of inquiry that permit an examination not only of conventional endpoints, such as survival, but also of others, such as pain control, that are of immediate relevance to patients.

References

1. Bruchovsky N, Wilson JD. The conversion of testosterone to 5′-androstan-17′-ol-3-one by rat prostate in vivo and in vitro. *J Biol Chem* 1968;243:2012-7.
2. Rennie PS, Bruchovsky N, Leco KJ, Sheppard PC, McQueen SA, Cheng H, et al. Characterization of two *cis*-acting DNA elements involved in the androgen regulation of the probasin gene. *Mol Endocrinol* 1993;7:23-36.
3. Huggins C, Hodges CV. Studies on prostatic cancer: I. The effect of castration, of estrogen and of androgen injection on serum phosphatases in metastatic carcinoma of the prostate. *Cancer Res* 1941;1:293-7.
4. Cox RL, Crawford ED. Estrogens in the treatment of prostate cancer. *J Urol* 1995;154:1991-8.
5. Leuprolide Study Group. Leuprolide versus diethylstilbestrol for metastatic prostate cancer. *N Engl J Med* 1984;311:1281-6.
6. Bruchovsky N. Androgens and antiandrogens. In: Holland JF, Frei E 3rd, Bast RC, Kufe DW, Morton DL, Weichselbaum RR, editors. *Cancer medicine*. 3rd ed. Philadelphia: Lea & Febiger; 1993. p. 884-96.
7. Blackledge GR. High-dose bicalutamide monotherapy for the treatment of prostate cancer. *Urology* 1996;47(1A Suppl):44-7.
8. Schellhammer PF, Sharifi R, Block N, Soloway MS, Venner PM, Patterson AM, et al. A controlled trial of bicalutamide vs flutamide, each in combination with LHRH analogue therapy, in patients with advanced prostate cancer. *Cancer* 1996;78:2164-9.
9. Goldenberg SL, Bruchovsky N, Gleave ME, Sullivan LD. Low-dose cyproterone acetate plus mini-dose diethylstilbestrol — a protocol for reversible medical castration. *Urology* 1996;47:882-4.
10. Crawford ED, Eisenberger MA, McLeod DG, Spalding JT, Benson R, Dorr FA, et al. A controlled trial of leuprolide with and without flutamide in prostatic carcinoma. *N Engl J Med* 1989;321:419-24.
11. Prostate Cancer Trialists' Collaborative Group. Maximum androgen blockade in advanced prostate cancer: an overview of 22 randomised trials with 3283 deaths in 5710 patients. *Lancet* 1995;346:265-9.
12. Gleave ME, Hsieh JT. Experimental animal models for prostate cancer. In: Lange P, Scher H, Ragavahn D, editors. *Genitourinary oncology*. New York: Lippincott; 1997. p. 367-78.
13. Bruchovsky N, Goldenberg SL, Akakura K, Rennie PS. LHRH agonists in prostate cancer: elimination of flare reaction by pretreatment with cyproterone acetate and low-dose diethylstilbestrol. *Cancer* 1993;72:1685-91.
14. Miller JI, Ahmann FR, Drach GW, Emerson SS, Bottaccini MR. The clinical usefulness of serum prostate specific antigen after hormonal therapy of metastatic

prostate cancer. *J Urol* 1992;147:956-61.
15. Newling DWW, Denis L, Vermeylen K. Orchiectomy versus goserelin and flutamide in the treatment of newly diagnosed metastatic prostate cancer: analysis of the criteria of evaluation used in the European Organization for Research and Treatment of Cancer — Genitourinary Group Study 30853. *Cancer* 1993;72:3793-8.
16. Huggins C, Scott WW. Bilateral adrenalectomy in prostate cancer. *Ann Surg* 1945;122:1031-41.
17. Crawford ED, Eisenberger M, McLeod DG, Wilding G, Blumenstein BA. Comparison of bilateral orchiectomy with or without flutamide for the treatment of patients with stage D2 adenocarcinoma of the prostate: results of NCI intergroup study 0105 (SWOG and ECOG) [abstract]. *Br J Urol* 1997;80:278.
18. Byar DP. Proceedings: The Veterans Administration Cooperative Urological Research Group's studies of cancer of the prostate. *Cancer* 1973;32:1126-30.
19. Gleave M, Bruchovsky N, Goldenberg SL, Rennie P. Intermittent androgen suppression for prostate cancer: rationale and clinical experience. *Eur Urol* 1998;34:37-41.
20. Bolla M, Gonzalez MD, Warde P, Dubois JB, Mirimanoff RO, Storme G, et al. Improved survival in patients with locally advanced prostate cancer treated with radiotherapy and goserelin. *N Engl J Med* 1997;337:295-300.
21. Medical Research Council Prostate Cancer Working Party Investigators Group. Immediate vs deferred treatment for advanced prostate cancer: initial results of the MRC trial. *Br J Urol* 1997;79:235-46.
22. Bruchovsky N, Goldenberg SL, Gleave ME, Rennie P, Akakura K, Sato N. Intermittent therapy for prostate cancer. *Endocr Rel Cancer* 1997;4:1-25.
23. Fleshner NE, Trachtenberg J. Combination finasteride and flutamide in advanced carcinoma of the prostate: effective theapy with minimal side effects. *J Urol* 1995;154:1642-6.
24. Siu LL, Moore MJ. Is there a role for chemotherapy in hormone refractory prostate cancer? *Adv Oncol* 1996;12:22-7.
25. Schmidt JD, Scott WW, Gibbons R, Johnson DE, Prout GR Jr, Loening S, et al. Chemotherapy programs of the National Prostate Cancer Project (NPCP). *Cancer* 1980;45:1937-46.
26. Moore MJ, Osoba D, Murphy K, Tannock IF, Armitage A, Findlay B, et al. Use of palliative end points to evaluate the effects of mitoxantrone and low-dose prednisone in patients with hormonally resistant prostate cancer. *J Clin Oncol* 1994;12:689-94.
27. Tannock IF, Osoba D, Stockler MR, Ernst DS, Neville AJ, Moore MF, et al. Chemotherapy with mitoxantrone plus prednisone or prednisone alone for symptomatic hormone-resistant prostate cancer: a Canadian randomized trial with palliative endpoints. *J Clin Oncol* 1996;14:1756-64.
28. Hudes GR, Greenberg R, Krigel RL, Fox S, Scher R, Litwin S, et al. Phase II study of estramustine and vinblastine, two microtubule inhibitors, in hormone-refractory prostate cancer. *J Clin Oncol* 1992;10:1754-61.
29. Pienta KJ, Redman B, Hussain M, Cummings G, Esper PS, Appel C, et al. Phase II evaluation of oral estramustine and oral etoposide in hormone-refractory adenocarcinoma of the prostate. *J Clin Oncol* 1994;12:2005-12.
30. Hudes GR, Nathan FE, Khater C, Haas N, Cornfield M, Giantonio B, et al. Phase II

trial of 96 hour paclitaxel plus estramustine in metastatic hormone-refractory prostate cancer. *J Clin Oncol* 1997;15:3156-63.

31. Myers C, Cooper M, Stein C, LaRocca R, Wlather MM, Weiss G, et al. Suramin: a novel growth factor antagonist with activity in hormone refractory metastatic prostate cancer. *J Clin Oncol* 1992;10:881-9.

32. Eisenberger MA, Reyno LM, Jodrell DI, Sinibaldi VJ, Tkaczuk KH, Sridhara R, et al. Suramin, an active drug for prostate cancer: interim observations in a phase I trial. *J Natl Cancer Inst* 1993;85:611-21.

33. Kelly WK, Curley T, Leibertz C, Dnistrian A, Schwartz M, Scher HI. Prospective evaluation of hydrocortisone and suramin in patients with androgen-independent prostate cancer. *J Clin Oncol* 1995;13:2208-13.

10

Palliative care

Neill A. Iscoe, MD, MSc; Eduardo Bruera, MD; Richard C. Choo, MD

> A 72-year-old man with no significant illnesses apart from his prostate cancer visits his urologist for follow-up. His prostate cancer was diagnosed 6 years earlier and was treated with radical local therapy. He was well for 3 years, then experienced relapse with bone metastases and pain. Treatment consisted of bilateral orchidectomy, and his symptoms were controlled for 24 months. As the disease progressed, anti-androgen therapy was started. However, over the past 6 months, the symptoms and level of disease, as indicated by prostate-specific antigen, have been increasing, despite withdrawal of the anti-androgen, spot irradiation and a regimen of cytotoxic chemotherapy. The patient is aware that his disease cannot be cured but wants to ask his physician about complementary therapies, such as green tea and Essiac, and he wants to know what more can be done for him.

The issues raised by the patient described in the case are understandable and altogether too common. He is aware that his prostate cancer cannot be cured with currently available treatments and is asking for care that will relieve his discomfort while he explores other, less conventional forms of treatment. In this article we provide an overview of complementary therapies (sometimes called unconventional or alternative therapies) and describe the current role of radiation therapy and palliative care in relation to the problems commonly encountered by men with progressive prostate cancer.

Complementary therapy

This particular patient has asked about green tea and Essiac, although he could just as easily have asked questions related to mind–body therapies, various diets or nutritional supplements, therapies that purport to augment the immune system and a host of other manoeuvres. The range of interventions is further confused by the terms used to describe them: unconventional, unorthodox, unproven, alternative and complementary. Although an Office of Technology Assessment report[1] to the United States Congress referred to these therapies as "unconventional," most proponents prefer the term "complementary," because they are often (although not uniformly) used to complement standard medical care.

> **KEY POINTS**
> - "Complementary" or "alternative" therapies are receiving more and more attention; however, most of these treatments, which cover a wide range of approaches, have not been subjected to any accepted medical testing protocol.
> - To assess these therapies, patients need to understand the standard criteria for evaluating an intervention and for attributing causation.
> - Because of the lack of evidence to support most complementary therapies, their use is often based solely on a belief that the treatment will improve disease control or well-being.

What physicians must realize is that this approach to care is exceedingly common. Although no accurate Canadian data are available, recent figures from the United States suggest that expenditures on these interventions increased substantially between 1990 and 1997 and that patients there now spend in excess of $21 billion annually on unconventional therapies for all disorders.[2] Patients seek complementary therapies for many reasons, including their need to assert some control over their situation, their belief system (which may differ from the physician's) and their need to examine their lives in the context of a life-threatening illness. Although the reasons why a patient seeks complementary therapies are of immense importance in understanding the patient's needs, they are not the subject of this chapter.

No one should dismiss a patient's desire to try anything that might provide greater disease control and comfort. Given the myriad of options from which patients may choose and the potential for unscrupulous people to take advantage of vulnerable patients, how is a practitioner to guide the patient in making an informed choice, if he is determined to seek out a complementary therapy?

These therapies may be promoted by physicians who have graduated from reputable medical schools as well as by people with no such training. Although the latter may be a cause for concern, the common feature of these therapies is that they have not been assessed by standard investigative methods. For some, such as homeopathic therapy, in which a noxious substance is administered in infinitely small dilutions, the underlying premise of the therapy defies the standard laws of physics. For others, the premise is either outside the accepted notions of biology or based on ideas that cannot be tested. Some therapies are based on a product whose composition is known only to its manufacturer and which has not been subjected to any inquiry into its physical or chemical nature.

How then does one advise desperate patients about the likelihood of a given intervention doing more harm than good? Although randomized controlled trials (RCTs), ideally of a double-blind nature, are the "gold standard" of assessment, the profession must acknowledge that many frequently used *conventional* therapies have not been subjected to this standard. Therefore, the presence or absence of an RCT should not be the sole criterion on which a decision is based. It may be useful to examine both the criteria for evaluating an intervention and those for attributing causation (i.e., the likelihood that exposure to a particular event will produce a given outcome) (Table 1).[3,4] Explaining these criteria to patients or their families in simple terms will probably give them the tools they need to make their own assessments. The essence of these recommendations is that patients should behave like consumers in this domain and should request from the prospective practitioner documentation that has been subjected to external scrutiny in support of the therapy in question.

For example, let us examine the situation in which a patient asks about second-line cytotoxic chemotherapy for prostate cancer and the use of a hypothetical unconventional therapy called etatsorp. Second-line cytotoxic chemotherapy has not been assessed in the treatment of prostate cancer, but it has been evaluated for other malignant diseases, for which defined response patterns and toxicity profiles are reported. Those promoting etatsorp claim that it relieves pain and controls the cancer by enhancing the immune system. The claimants suggest

Table 1: Criteria for evaluating reports of an intervention and attributing causation*

Evaluating reports of an intervention
Were subjects assigned randomly to receive the intervention?
Were all clinically important outcomes reported?
Were the study patients similar to your own?
Were both clinical and statistical significance considered?
Is the intervention feasible in your practice?
Were all patients accounted for at the end of the study?

Attributing causation
Is there a true experiment in humans?
Is the association strong?
Is the association consistent between studies of the same question?
Is the temporal relation correct?
Is there a dose–response relation?
Is the association epidemiologically sensible?
Does the association make sense biologically?
Is the association specific?
Is the association analogous to a previously proven causal association?

*Adapted from *CMAJ* with permission.[3,4]

> **KEY POINTS**
> - Radiotherapy has been the mainstay in the palliation of symptomatic metastatic prostate cancer.
> - Treatment may consist of external-beam radiotherapy (local-field or hemibody irradiation) or systemic radionuclides (e.g., strontium 89).
> - Radiotherapy is used for palliation of
>   - painful bone metastases
>   - spinal cord or nerve root compression
>   - symptoms caused by the local progression of prostate cancer
>   - mass effect of metastatic lymphadenopathy.

that these effects occur in all cancers to some extent, but that this agent is particularly effective in prostate cancer. The proponents argue that etatsorp is most useful when the burden of disease is small and, therefore, that patients should use it as soon as possible after diagnosis. Although personal testimonials are offered, there is no standard medical documentation of these cases.

With reference to the criteria in Table 1, it is apparent that neither cytotoxic chemotherapy nor etatsorp has been subjected to trials assessing its activity in the management of patients with prostate cancer; similarly, there have been no RCTs to compare their effectiveness with that of other therapies or best supportive care. RCTs of the cytotoxic agent are foreseeable, and claims that RCTs for complementary therapies are impossible — because each patient is unique — are invalid.[5] Therefore, the patient's decision about using these methods must be based on inference and beliefs rather than on evidence.

In this example the criteria related to causation are most helpful in decision-making. Is there a biological rationale for the therapy, and are there analogous situations in which the agent has been objectively evaluated and its activity or efficacy documented? In the case of standard chemotherapy there is a biological basis for believing that the therapy has the *potential* to produce a response. However, second-line chemotherapy invariably has less activity against malignant disease than first-line therapy, and first-line chemotherapy in prostate cancer has limited activity. Therefore, although there may be a biological basis supporting this therapy, in reality there should be little optimism that it will be effective for patients with prostate cancer.

In the hypothetical example, etatsorp is purported to be an enhancer of the immune system. The extent to which this statement is supported by documented objective and, perhaps, reproducible in-vivo or in-vitro evidence is critical in determining its potential merit. It must also be determined whether an objective benefit has been noted in clinical situations sufficiently analogous to our patient's to provide a foundation for considering the treatment. Unfortunately, because most complementary therapies are developed outside the usual investigational models, the background information to support or refute the premise is seldom available. Perhaps more distressing is the same dearth of information at the clinical level.

As physicians, we should warn this man that complementary therapies can be expensive, that imported compounds may not be produced under safe and acceptable conditions, and that other countries may not require labelling even though the compounds contain powerful agents.

Therefore, the advice to this patient should be that the only reason to pursue either cytotoxic therapy or etatsorp therapy is a *belief* that the treatment will work, since there is no evidence in favour of the use of either. Whatever transpires, the physician should continue to provide support and comfort to the patient and his family through this difficult time.

Palliative radiotherapy

Radiotherapy has been a mainstay in the palliation of symptomatic metastatic prostate cancer and is most often used for palliation of painful metastatic bone lesions. Other medical problems amenable to palliative radiotherapy include compression of the spinal cord or a nerve root, hematuria, ureteric obstruction, and perineal discomfort caused by the local progression of prostate cancer and symptomatic metastatic lymphadenopathy.

Skeletal metastatic lesions

The most common symptom in metastatic prostate cancer is pain from bone lesions, particularly in the spine and pelvis. Palliative radiotherapy is usually indicated unless pain is relieved by well-tolerated analgesics. In general, 80% to 90% of patients obtain some degree of pain relief from palliative radiotherapy. In addition to pain relief, the goals of this treatment include elimination or reduction of the need for narcotics and arrest of local tumour growth that might otherwise lead to compression of the spinal cord or pathologic fracture.

Palliative radiotherapy for bone metastases may consist of local-field radiotherapy, hemibody irradiation or use of systemic radionuclides. Local-field and hemibody treatments are delivered by external-beam irradiation, whereas systemic radionuclide therapy is given intravenously, by means of bone-seeking radioactive isotopes. Factors to be considered in the selection of the radiation modality and the extent of radiation therapy for an individual patient include estimated life expectancy, functional status, bone marrow function, extent and volume of metastatic bone lesions, number of symptomatic sites, presence of visceral metastasis and previous treatments.

Local-field radiotherapy

Patients with several metastatic bone lesions, only one or a few of which are symptomatic, can be effectively treated with local-field external-beam irradiation (Fig. 1). Pain flare may occur in some patients at the beginning of radiotherapy. This usually lasts 2–3 days and generally predicts a good palliative response. Pain relief usually begins 1–2 weeks after the start of therapy and invariably is present, if it occurs at all, within 1–3 months. Imaging studies that correlate with the signs and symptoms of bone metastasis aid in designing the radiation field. Local-field irradiation is generally well tolerated and has minimal acute toxic effects and negligible long-term adverse effects.

Several prospective randomized trials and retrospective studies have suggested that high-dose, protracted palliative radiotherapy delivered over a lengthy period of time has no consistent advantage over single-dose or low-dose short-course regimens.[6–11] For a debilitated patient with a short life expectancy, for whom daily trips for fractionated treatment would be burdensome, it is appropriate and expedient to give single-fraction irradiation. On the other hand, a more fractionated higher-dose regimen is generally used for patients with one or a few sites of metastasis who have good functional status and reasonable life expectancy.

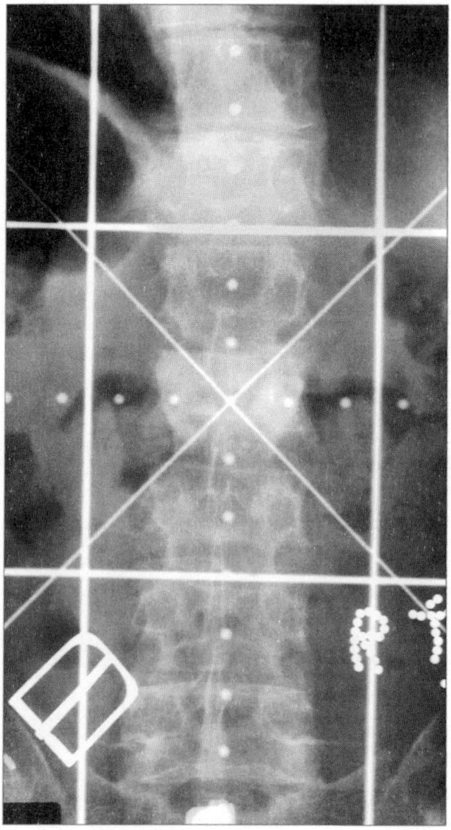

Hemibody irradiation

Hemibody irradiation involves delivering radiation in single or multiple fractions to a large volume of tissue (Fig. 2). It has been used for patients with many painful metastatic bone lesions who have adequate bone marrow function, as an alternative to a series of local-field irradiation doses directed at specific painful sites. Its main purpose is to avoid repeated trips to the hospital for multiple courses of irradiation.

Improved pain control has been reported in up to 80% of patients treated with single-fraction irradiation to the upper or lower half-body.[12–14] Irradiation to the lower or mid-body is generally well tolerated if pretreatment medication is given to minimize nausea and vomiting.

Fig. 1: Simulation radiograph demonstrating local-field radiotherapy of the spine. The rectangular area delimited by the white lines represents the irradiated volume of tissue.

Upper half-body irradiation is generally associated with more severe side effects, which often necessitate a day in hospital, hydration, and premedication with antiemetics and corticosteroids.

Systemic radionuclide therapy

Radioactive isotopes, administered intravenously, have been used to palliate pain from widespread metastatic bone lesions. Strontium 89 is the injectable, nonsealed radionuclide most commonly used for hormone-refractory metastatic prostate cancer. Although it is preferentially taken up and retained by sites of osteoblastic metastases, it is washed out of healthy bone, where its biological half-life is 14 days.[15,16] This differential distribution and retention of the nuclide results in preferential delivery of radiation to metastatic sites and therefore therapeutic gain.

On the basis of results from several RCTs,[16–19] ^{89}Sr is generally recommended for patients with many metastatic bone lesions associated with uncontrolled pain on both sides of the diaphragm, for whom the use of multiple single fields of external-beam radiotherapy is difficult and impractical. In one trial, lessening of pain was observed in 70% of the patients.[16] This agent has also been used in conjunction with local-field radiotherapy for patients with isolated painful metastatic lesions. In this clinical setting, it can delay, by up to 15 weeks, the need for further radiotherapy at new painful sites and can temporarily reduce the intake of analgesics.[19] However, the clinical significance of these benefits is uncertain. Pain flare occurs in a small proportion of patients and generally lasts 2–4 days. Pain relief usually begins in 2–3 weeks, with maximal relief and nadir blood counts at 6 weeks.

The main side effect of ^{89}Sr is suppression of bone marrow function. Because a patient may already have a reduced reserve of bone marrow as a result of previous

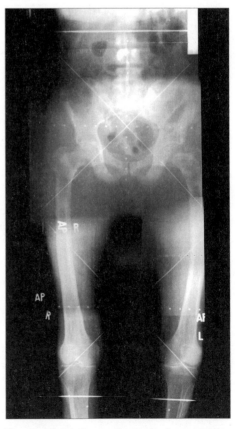

Fig. 2: Simulation radiograph demonstrating hemibody irradiation to the lower half-body. In this case the area irradiated extends from about the waist to just below the knees.

external-beam radiotherapy, myelosuppressive chemotherapy or tumour infiltration of the bone marrow, it is imperative to assess carefully the patient's eligibility for ^{89}Sr treatment. Systemic radionuclide therapy is not recommended for those with inadequate bone marrow reserves or inadequate renal function, nor for patients whose main symptomatic lesions show inadequate uptake on bone scanning. It is also contraindicated as the sole treatment in patients with fracture or impending fracture and compression of the spinal cord or a nerve root. Because ^{89}Sr is a β emitter and is excreted in the urine, its use in men who are incontinent or who have indwelling catheters poses greater radiation safety concerns and is thus contraindicated.[20] ^{89}Sr must be administered in the appropriate context and only after an evaluation of the patient's overall status, previous therapy and possible future treatments, so an oncologist with expertise in the overall management of prostate cancer should be involved in its use.

Compression of the spinal cord or a nerve root

In cases of metastatic disease compromising the integrity of the spinal cord or a nerve root, urgent intervention is required to minimize neurological dysfunction. Pain is the most common presenting symptom and generally precedes neurological deficit. Magnetic resonance imaging of the spine or myelography with computed tomography at the level where compression is suspected is essential to identify all levels of blockage.

Palliative radiotherapy, either alone or as an adjunct to surgical decompression, is usually indicated for managing compression of the spinal cord or a nerve root. Surgical decompression should be considered in patients with significant pathologic compression of vertebrae, instability of the spine, neurological deterioration during radiotherapy or compression at a previously irradiated site. A short course of fractionated radiotherapy is often effective for relieving pain and reversing neurological dysfunction. In a recent series of 50 patients treated with external-beam radiation, 67% had neurological improvement and 92% experienced pain relief.[21]

The primary determinant of neurological recovery after any form of therapy for spinal cord compression is neurological status and duration of neurological deficit before the intervention. Thus, prompt diagnosis, evaluation and treatment are essential to reverse any existing deficits and to preserve maximum function.

Other indications

Palliative radiotherapy is effective in relieving symptoms secondary to the local progression of prostate cancer, such as hematuria, ureteric obstruction and perineal pain. It is also beneficial for patients with leg edema or back discomfort caused by metastatic pelvic or para-aortic lymphadenopathy. Similarly, any clinical symptoms related to tumour mass effect can be palliated with radiotherapy.

Symptom control

The patient described at the outset of this article already has bone pain. Although this pain may be relieved by radiation therapy, seldom will such treatment control the symptoms of metastatic bone lesions until death. The management of pain and the control of other symptoms become paramount in caring for this man (Table 2).

Table 2: Symptom control in prostate cancer

Symptom	Suggested therapy
Pain	Opioid analgesics (oral or subcutaneous) Radiation therapy Bisphosphonates
Gastrointestinal symptoms	Megestrol acetate Corticosteroids Metoclopramide Laxatives
Delirium	Regular monitoring of cognition Opioid rotation Methadone Haloperidol

Pain

This patient has pain because of metastatic bone lesions. Continuous bone pain responds well to opioid analgesics. Most patients will experience good analgesia with a combination of acetaminophen plus codeine or oxycodone. After several weeks or months, this man will likely require stronger opioid agonists such as morphine or hydromorphone (drugs with similar effectiveness and toxicity).[22] The initiation of opioid analgesics represents a major hurdle for some patients, in terms of fears of addiction or uncontrolled pain and the symbolic message that their illness has become serious enough that such agents are necessary. Physicians should be aware of these concerns and address them directly. In particular they should reassure patients that addiction is not an issue and that adequate pain control can be achieved in most cases. Patients should always undergo titration to good pain control with short-acting opioids every 4 hours before being switched over to a maintenance dose of a slow-release opioid preparation. Slow-release preparations of morphine (once or twice a day), hydromorphone, codeine, oxycodone and fentanyl (transdermal patches every 3 days) are currently available in Canada. Patients receiving long- or short-acting opioids should have access to extra doses of approximately 10% of the total daily opioid dose for episodes of more severe pain.

Before death, about 80% of patients will require an alternative route of opioid administration for periods ranging from hours to months. The subcutaneous route allows patients to receive analgesia safely and effectively at home as intermittent injections into a butterfly needle every 4 hours from preloaded syringes or low-cost devices such as the Edmonton Injector.[23] A small proportion of patients may require a more expensive device for subcutaneous infusion of opioids.

As previously discussed, radiation therapy can relieve bone pain in 80% to 90% of patients and should be considered for all patients who experience pain in the long bones or for those with a single or predominant painful area.

Bisphosphonates can be administered as an intravenous infusion (pamidronate or clodronate) or as a subcutaneous infusion (clodronate) to decrease generalized bone pain and prevent osteolysis. An infusion every 3–4 weeks over 4 hours can reduce the need for opioid analgesics and radiation therapy and decrease the number of bone fractures.[24,25] The evidence for benefit from bisphosphonates is greater in breast cancer and melanoma. However, at least one study found significant improvement in prostate cancer.[24]

Approximately 20% of patients with metastatic bone lesions have minimal or no pain if they remain completely immobile but experience severe "incidental" pain when they move.[26] In this situation, pain control may be difficult, and patients should be referred to a palliative care or pain specialist.

Gastrointestinal symptoms

The patient described at the beginning of this article will probably experience progressive severe anorexia. Numerous studies have shown that megestrol acetate can be used to treat anorexia, improve food intake, reduce fatigue and produce a sensation of well-being. The effects become evident after 1–2 weeks of treatment.[27] Because progestational drugs must be used at doses ranging from 3 to 5 times the antineoplastic dose (e.g., the dose of megestrol acetate would be 480–800 mg/d), these drugs can be quite expensive. Corticosteroids are also effective appetite stimulants. They are inexpensive and also have antinausea and analgesic effects. However, they do not lead to increased food intake or weight gain, and their effect is short lived (usually less than 4 weeks). The most effective type, dose and route of administration of corticosteroids have not been established. In summary, ambulatory patients with good performance status who complain of profound anorexia could be given a brief course of megestrol acetate. On the other hand, patients whose condition has deteriorated severely and who have severe pain and nausea might benefit from a course of oral or subcutaneous corticosteroids.

Chronic nausea is almost universal in patients with advanced prostate cancer. It results from a combination of autonomic failure with resulting gastroparesis due to advanced cancer, cachexia, opioid therapy, constipation and metabolic abnormalities. Short-acting metoclopramide (10–20 mg every 4 hours) or long-acting metoclopramide (every 12 hours) alone or in combination with corticosteroids and aggressive laxative therapy can be used to control this symptom in most patients.

Finally, constipation is a highly prevalent and underdiagnosed symptom capable of aggravating abdominal pain and causing anorexia, nausea and urinary retention in these patients. All patients with advanced prostate cancer should receive regular oral laxatives, and the frequency and type of bowel movements should be monitored regularly.

> **KEY POINTS**
> - Other symptoms of advanced prostate cancer include severe pain, gastrointestinal problems and delirium. A variety of simple measures can be used to address each of these problems.
> - Although at this stage it may be impossible to treat the disease, much can be done to ensure the patient's comfort as his disease progresses. Attending to a patient's needs may require referral to other physicians or the involvement of a variety of other health care professionals.

Delirium

More than 85% of patients with prostate cancer will experience progressive confusion before death.[28] In these usually elderly patients, the delirium results from many factors. The most frequent reasons are opioid analgesics, psychoactive drugs, sepsis, dehydration, renal failure and other metabolic abnormalities. Brain metastases are rare in patients with prostate cancer.

Approximately a third of episodes of delirium are fully reversible with simple measures such as opioid rotation (a change in opioid type), hydration, antibiotic therapy or discontinuation of psychoactive drugs.[28]

Opioids should always be considered a potential contributing factor in delirium. This effect is mainly due to the accumulation of active opioid metabolite in patients receiving high doses or undergoing prolonged treatment and in those who have renal failure or dehydration of recent onset. Opioid-induced delirium is frequently associated with generalized myoclonus, agitation, hyperalgesia and tactile hallucinations.[29] Rotation to another opioid allows the active metabolites to be eliminated, usually within 48 hours. The opioid should be used at lower equi-analgesic dose and titrated cautiously. Delirium has been observed with all opioid agonists, including morphine, hydromorphone, meperidine, codeine, oxycodone and fentanyl. In patients who present with rapid dose escalation or repeated episodes of opioid-induced delirium, rotation to methadone may be considered. This synthetic agonist has the advantages of extremely low cost and absence of active metabolites. However, the dose ratio between methadone and other opioids is not well known, and there is the potential for severe toxic effects. Therefore, rotation to methadone should be undertaken only by an experienced palliative care cancer or pain specialist.

Approximately a third of patients with delirium present with severe psychomotor agitation, hallucination or delusional thoughts. In these patients, haloperidol should be administered regularly, by oral or subcutaneous route, for 1 or 2 days while investigation or management of the delirium is implemented. In extreme cases, sedation, by continuous subcutaneous infusion of midazolam, may be required.

Conclusions

For the patient described in the case at the beginning of this article, there may not be a great deal that medicine can do to control his disease generally. This article has focused only on the medical management of selected problems encountered by men with prostate cancer and their families. Depending on individual circumstances, other physicians may be helpful in managing symptomatic problems, for example, orthopedic surgeons for skeletal problems. More important, physicians should not forget others, such as religious leaders, nutritionists, physiotherapists, psychologists and occupational therapists, who may provide valuable advice and comfort for patients. Finally, our experience is that most patients wish to remain at home for as long as possible. The integration of their care in community hospice and palliative care programs at the earliest opportunity will assist in achieving the seamless care desired and will mimimize the potential for the crisis situations that commonly occur when such aspects are not considered in the patient's care. Much can be done to provide comfort for this man as his disease progresses over the ensuing months. The most important thing to remember is that care not only remains possible, but now assumes even greater importance in the absence of effective therapies that can be directed at his cancer.

References

1. Office of Technology Assessment. *Unconventional cancer treatments*. Washington: United States Government Printing Office; 1990. Rep no. OTA-H-405.
2. Eisenberg DM, Davis RB, Ettner SL, Appel S, Wilkey S, Van Rompay M, et al. Trends in alternative medicine use in the United States, 1990–1997. Results of a follow-up national survey. *JAMA* 1998;280:1569-75.
3. Department of Clinical Epidemiology and Biostatistics, McMaster University Health Sciences Centre. How to read clinical journals: IV. To determine etiology or causation. *CMAJ* 1981;124:985-90.
4. Department of Clinical Epidemiology and Biostatistics, McMaster University Health Sciences Centre. How to read clinical journals: V. To distinguish useful from useless or even harmful therapy. *CMAJ* 1981;124:1156-62.
5. Fontanarosa PB, Lundberg GD. Alternative medicine meets science [editorial]. *JAMA*

1998;280:1618-9.
6. Cole DJ. A randomized trial of a single treatment versus conventional fractionation in the palliative radiotherapy of painful bone metastases. *Clin Oncol* 1989;1:59-62.
7. Madsen EL. Painful bone metastasis: efficacy of radiotherapy assessed by the patients: a randomized trial comparing 4 Gy × 6 versus 10 Gy × 2. *Int J Radiat Oncol Biol Phys* 1983;9:1775-9.
8. Price P, Hoskin PJ, Easton D, Austin D, Palmer SG, Yarnold JR. Prospective randomised trial of single and multifraction radiotherapy schedules in the treatment of painful bony metastases. *Radiother Oncol* 1986;6:247-55.
9. Tong D, Gillick L, Hendrickson FR. The palliation of symptomatic osseous metastases: final results of the study by the Radiation Therapy Oncology Group. *Cancer* 1982;50:893-9.
10. Blitzer PH. Reanalysis of the RTOG study of the palliation of symptomatic osseous metastasis. *Cancer* 1985;55:1468-72.
11. Arcangeli G, Micheli A, Arcangeli G, Giannarelli D, La Pasta O, Tollis A, et al. The responsiveness of bone metastases to radiotherapy: the effect of site, histology and radiation dose on pain relief. *Radiother Oncol* 1989;14:95-101.
12. Fitzpatrick PJ, Rider WD. Half-body radiotherapy. *Int J Radiat Oncol Biol Phys* 1976;1:197-207.
13. Salazar OM, Rubin P, Hendrickson FR, Poulter C, Zagars G, Feldman MI, et al. Single-dose half-body irradiation for the palliation of multiple bone metastases from solid tumors: a preliminary report. *Int J Radiat Oncol Biol Phys* 1981;7:773-81.
14. Zelefsky MJ, Scher HI, Forman JD, Linares LA, Curley T, Fuks Z. Palliative hemiskeletal irradiation for widespread metastatic prostate cancer: a comparison of single dose and fractionated regimens. *Int J Radiat Oncol Biol Phys* 1989;17:1281-5.
15. Ben-Josef E, Lucas DR, Vasan S, Porter AT. Selective accumulation of strontium-89 in metastatic deposits in bone: radio-histological correlation. *Nucl Med Commun* 1995;16:457-63.
16. Quilty PM, Kirk D, Bolger JJ, Dearnaley DP, Lewington VJ, Mason MD, et al. A comparison of the palliative effects of strontium-89 and external beam radiotherapy in metastatic prostate cancer. *Radiother Oncol* 1994;31:33-40.
17. Lewington VJ, McEwan AJ, Ackery DM, Bayly RJ, Keeling DH, Macleod PM, et al. A prospective, randomized double-blind crossover study to examine the efficacy of strontium-89 in pain palliation in patients with advanced prostate cancer metastatic to bone. *Eur J Cancer* 1991;27:954-8.
18. Buchali K, Correns HJ, Schuerer M, Schnoor D, Lips H, Sydow K. Results of a double blind study of 89-strontium therapy of skeletal metastases of prostatic carcinoma. *Eur J Nucl Med* 1988;14:349-51.
19. Porter AT, McEwan AJ, Powe JE, Reid R, McGowan DG, Lukka H, et al. Results of a randomized phase-III trial to evaluate the efficacy of strontium-89 adjuvant to local field external beam irradiation in the management of endocrine resistant metastatic prostate cancer. *Int J Radiat Oncol Biol Phys* 1993;25:805-13.
20. Porter AT, Ben-Josef E. Strontium 89 in the treatment of bone metastases. In: DeVita VT, Helman S, Rosenberg SA, editors. *Important advances in oncology*. Philadelphia: JB Lippincott; 1995. p. 87-94.
21. Zelefsky JM, Scher HI, Krol G, Portenoy RK, Leibel SA, Fuks ZY. Spinal epidural tumor in patients with prostate cancer. *Cancer* 1992;70:2319-25.

22. Management of cancer pain: clinical practice guidelines. Rockville (MD): Agency for Health Care Policy and Research, Department of Health and Human Services; 1994. AHCPR publ 94-0592.
23. Bruera E, Valasco-Leiva A, Spachynski K, Fainsinger R, Miller MJ, MacEachern T. The use of the Edmonton Injector (EI) for parenteral opioid management of cancer pain: a study of 100 consecutive patients. *J Pain Symptom Manage* 1993;8:525-8.
24. Bloomfield DJ. Should bisphosphonates be part of standard therapy of patients with multiple myeloma and bone metastases from other cancers? An evidence-based review. *J Clin Oncol* 1998;16:1218-26.
25. Ernst DS, Brasher P, Hagen N, Paterson AHG, MacDonald RN, Bruera E. A randomized, controlled trial of intravenous clodronate in patients with metastatic bone disease and pain. *J Pain Symptom Manage* 1997;13:319-26.
26. Bruera E, Schoeller T, Wenk R, MacEachern T, Marcelino S, Suarez-Almazor M, et al. A prospective multi-center assessment of the Edmonton Staging System for cancer pain. *J Pain Symptom Manage* 1995;10:348-55.
27. Fainsinger R. Pharmacological approach to cancer anorexia and cachexia. In: Bruera E, Higginson L, editors. *Cachexia–anorexia in cancer patients*. Oxford: Oxford University Press; 1996. p. 128-40.
28. Pereira J, Hanson J, Bruera E. The frequency and clinical course of cognitive impairment in patients with terminal cancer. *Cancer* 1997;79:835-42.
29. Ripamonti C, Bruera E. CNS adverse effects of opioids in cancer patients. Guidelines for treatment. *Cent Nerv Syst Drugs* 1997;8:21-37.

11

Alternative approaches and the future of treatment

John Trachtenberg, MD; Juanita Crook, MD; Ian F. Tannock, MD, PhD

> A 72-year-old man with a family history of prostate cancer was treated for this disease by radical surgery 5 years ago. He has been well since but has seen friends experience relaspe and die after initial treatment with surgery or radiation and subsequent drug therapy. He is aware that his sons are at increased risk for prostate cancer and asks his physician what treatments are likely to be available in the future.

Prostate cancer is a leading cause of cancer deaths in men. No study has demonstrated that any particular treatment prolongs overall survival beyond what would be expected if no treatment was given. However, several studies have demonstrated that, if no treatment is undertaken, patients with moderate or high-grade prostate cancer and those with any grade of prostate cancer whose life expectancy is more than 10 years have a substantially shorter life span than men who do not have prostate cancer. Thus, most clinicians accept that selected patients will experience benefit as a result of curative treatment for prostate cancer. Furthermore, there is a considerable body of evidence for the effectiveness of different treatments in eliminating prostate cancer and prolonging cancer-free survival. In this article we discuss recent advances in surgical treatment of prostate cancer, 2 new methods of administering radiotherapy and recent developments in treatment for hormone-refractory prostate cancer.

Future surgical alternatives

The ideal treatment for localized prostate cancer remains to be determined. Most urologic surgeons believe that radical prostatectomy is the best choice for men with a life expectancy of at least 15 years and in whom the cancer is apparently localized within the prostate, is moderately or poorly differentiated and is of small to moderate volume. This belief is based on the fact that only prostatectomy offers the possibility of complete excision of the tumour. Pathological assessment of the resected specimen can be used to confirm whether excision is complete and to determine whether early adjunctive therapy might be appropriate. Prostatectomy allows for the immediate and continuous use of a biological marker, prostate-specific antigen (PSA), to monitor the success of treatment: PSA should be undetectable within a month after the procedure and should remain so. These observations have been bolstered by the high rate of biochemical failure (30% to 70%, determined by PSA level) associated with the only other accepted means of curing prostate cancer — traditional external-beam radiation therapy. Furthermore, changes in the selection of patients and the conduct of radical prostatectomy have increased its success and minimized both the complications and the costs of the procedure.[1]

> **KEY POINTS**
> - Most urologists believe that radical prostatectomy offers the best opportunity for cure in selected patients.
> - Minimally invasive treatments are now being developed that may offer the advantages of surgery with few of its complications.
> - Interstitial microwave thermoablation, a still-experimental technique, involves implanting many small heat sources in the prostate to destroy localized cancer while preserving surrounding tissues.

In spite of these advantages, alternative surgical therapies have been developed to avoid the invasiveness and complications of radical prostatectomy, especially in difficult circumstances such as salvage after failed radiation therapy. The most commonly practised of these alternatives is cryosurgery. However, after its initial enthusiastic adoption, the use of this technique has declined markedly because of a high failure rate coupled with unacceptable side effects.[2,3]

Thermoablation of the prostate, by means of a variety of heat sources including laser, radio-frequency electromagnetic radiation, focused ultrasound and microwave energy, is another recent development.[4,5] The aim of this type of intervention is to ablate portions of the prostate surrounding the urethra and thus decrease urethral resistance. Various treatment protocols for thermoablation have met with different degrees of success.

Technological advances have allowed the development of one such treatment protocol, a minimally invasive surgical technique that offers many of the advantages of radical prostatectomy without the side effects. This technique, called interstitial microwave thermoablation, is performed by a team of urologists, medical imagers, physicists and computer experts and uses thermal energy to ablate the prostate through a percutaneous transperineal approach in a single outpatient session. This method has shown particular promise for patients in whom primary radiation therapy has failed. The heat source, which consists of a series of antennas 1.2 mm in diameter that radiate microwave energy of 912 MHz, is implanted in the prostate (Fig. 1). The theoretical ellipse-shaped heating pattern of each antenna is 3 × 2 cm. Pretreatment ultrasonography in conjunction with a 3-dimensional computer-assisted appraisal of volume and tissue consistency is used to determine the best placement sites for the antennas to ensure that the entire prostate is heated. Actual placement of the antennas is guided by transrectal ultrasonography and a template system.

The target temperature at the periphery of the gland (where the temperature will be lowest) is 60°C, and this temperature is maintained for 15 minutes. This temperature is believed adequate to completely destroy all viable cancer tissue. A small zone of urethral tissue is preserved by cooling the urethra. Although the prostate can easily be heated to very high temperatures, the surrounding tissues, such as the rectum and the penile neurovascular bundles, may be damaged by the heat applied to the prostate. To prevent harm to these structures, the technique of hydrodissection was developed. Fluid is infused into the virtual space between the prostate and the rectum, separating these structures. The fluid acts as insulation, allowing constant measurement of the interface temperature and, if necessary, active cooling of the space (Fig. 2).

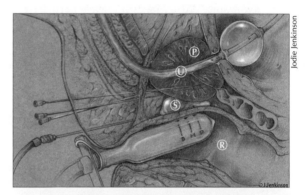

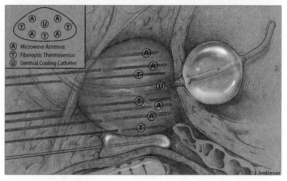

Fig. 1: Placement of microwave antennas in the prostate under ultrasound guidance for interstitial microwave thermoablation (top) and anatomic appearance during heating (bottom). The top image shows a hydrodissection space (S) between the prostate (P) and the rectum (R). A cooling catheter lies in the urethra (U).

Finally, online thermal imaging using phase-shift magnetic resonance imaging (MRI) has been developed to determine the actual temperature and thus to confirm that the target temperature has been reached in the prostate and that the temperature in the surrounding structures remains at a safe level.

We have used interstitial microwave thermoablation to treat a series of patients in whom primary radiation therapy for localized prostate cancer had failed (J.T., unpublished data). Recurrence of disease was documented by rising PSA levels and prostatic biopsy, and pretreatment evaluations failed to demonstrate any evidence of extraprostatic disease. We have at least 1 year of follow-up data for 13 patients whose pretreatment PSA level was less than 10 ng/mL. In 7 of these patients, the PSA level was undetectable and biopsy results were negative at 1 year (the biopsies showed only fibrous tissue with no recognizable prostatic elements). Post-treatment Doppler flow studies and gadolium-enhanced MRI in these patients suggested an absence of vascularization in what had been the prostate.

The side-effect profile of interstitial microwave thermoablation has been favourable. All patients reported perineal discomfort that could be treated with simple analgesics and that spontaneously dissipated by 1 month. There were no cases of fistulae or incontinence. The procedure can be done on an outpatient basis, although it does require general or spinal anesthesia.

Undoubtably, microwave thermoablation requires further refinement and evaluation, and it should be considered experimental. At present, it is limited to patients in whom radiation therapy has failed, in whom the residual prostate tumour is of small volume (preferably with a PSA level of less than 20 ng/mL), in whom there is no evidence of extraprostatic extension and who wish to be part of the trial at The Toronto Hospital. Nonetheless, the favourable early results are encouraging.[6,7] If future results continue to follow this trend, it might be reasonable to consider this technique as primary therapy in selected men. Interstitial microwave thermoablation offers a glimpse into the future, when total ablation of the prostate may

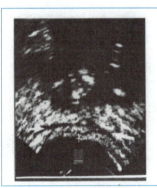
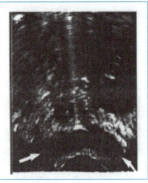

Fig. 2: Transrectal ultrasound images before (left) and after (right) infusion of fluid into the hydrodissection space. In the left-hand image, the arrows indicate a virtual space between the rectum and the prostate. In the right-hand image, the arrows point to the large space separating the rectum from the prostate, created by hydrodissection.

be accomplished rapidly, safely, effectively, inexpensively and in a minimally invasive manner.

Trends in radiotherapy

Localized prostate cancer is a radiocurable disease, and recent data stratifying patients by PSA level, stage and Gleason score have levelled the playing field for comparisons of the results of surgery and radiotherapy.[8] However, 2 main factors have in the past contributed to local failure after standard radiotherapy:
- inability to deliver sufficient radiation dose to the prostate because of the radiosensitivity of the adjacent rectum and bladder
- inability to shape the radiation field to the anatomic shape of the target.

These 2 problems are clearly linked, and recent advances in imaging and in treatment planning software, in the form of 2 new delivery systems for radiotherapy, have gone a long way toward solving them. Three-dimensional conformal radiotherapy relies on external treatment beams but improves markedly the ability to shape the beams and focus treatment on the prostate while avoiding the nearby bladder and rectum.[9] Interstitial brachytherapy involves the placement of radioactive seeds directly into the prostate to deliver the maximum dose to the prostate with a rapid decrease in dose through the rectum and bladder. Because both innovations address the problem of focusing radiation on the prostate, they permit safe delivery of a higher dose than would otherwise be possible. Although both are widely available in the United States, their use in Canada is still limited.

Conformal radiotherapy

The goal of conformal radiotherapy is to manipulate the distribution of the radiation dose so that it conforms to the shape of the target in 3 dimensions, thus minimizing the risk of missing or underdosing the target and maximizing the exclusion of normal tissue from the high-dose volume.[10]

A planning computed tomography (CT) scan is obtained with the patient in the treatment position and immobilized in a customized cradle or shell to maximize the reproducibility of his position and to minimize daily set-up variation during the subsequent course of treatment. CT slices are obtained at 5-mm intervals through the prostate and seminal vesicles. From these images, the contours of each organ of interest (the prostate, the seminal vesicles, the rectum and the bladder) are digitized and input into the treatment planning system.

The computer program reconstructs the patient's internal anatomy in 3 dimensions and can then rotate the reconstruction in an infinite variety of ways to determine the optimal angles for beam entry and the optimal shielding

> **KEY POINTS**
> - Radiotherapy for localized prostate cancer has been limited by physicians' inability to deliver a sufficient dose of radiation to the prostate without damaging adjacent organs.
> - Advances in computer-controlled radiotherapy allow consecutive scanning of target tissue, shaping of the beam to the desired form, and treatment, all within a fraction of the time usually required.
> - Improved imaging sytems are increasing the effectiveness of brachytherapy: in a procedure guided by transrectal ultrasonography, needles are used to implant strings of radioactive seeds in the prostate.

of normal structures. A margin (usually 1 cm or less) must be added to the volume delineated by the CT scans to account for possible extracapsular spread, motion of the target organs within the patient and set-up variation. The treatment is then simulated according to the computer-generated plan and verified by fluoroscopy.

Customized shielding is constructed to shape each treatment beam to the anatomic target. The shielding decreases the total volume treated by as much as 40% without compromising coverage of the target and reduces the toxic effects so that doses higher than the customary 66 Gy (i.e., 76–80 Gy) can be delivered safely.

The technology exists to streamline this process so that the CT scanning and simulation are done in one suite with a single machine, a CT simulator. This instrument acquires the transverse images at 5-mm intervals, then digitally reconstructs the classic orthogonal simulator "port films," superimposing the target volume, the adjacent organs of interest and the desired shaped radiation fields.

In the past, radiation beams were defined by a standard straight collimator jaw on the machine head. To shape the beam into any form other than a rectangle or a square, customized lead-alloy shielding blocks had to be constructed for each patient and placed manually into the beam at the time of each treatment. Now, new multileaf collimators replace the standard straight collimator jaw with dozens of tiny independent segments that can be opened or closed to various degrees under computer control to achieve any field shape.

During computer-controlled radiotherapy, once the patient is positioned and immobilized on the treatment table, the linear accelerator head rotates around the patient, stopping at each predetermined beam-entry angle, shapes each beam to the desired form, administers the radiation and moves on to the next position, without the technologists having to re-enter the room, manually rotate the machine or change shielding blocks for each beam. Despite the increased complexity, the treatment can be completed in a fraction of the time of conventional external-beam radiotherapy.

Brachytherapy

Implantation of radioactive seeds in the prostate using an open but freehand suprapubic approach was popular in the late 1970s and early 1980s. The early results seemed satisfactory, with good local tumour control and minimal bladder or sexual sequelae. However, because of the inherent inhomogeneity of the freehand implantation, the long-term results were disappointing, and prostate brachytherapy became unpopular for several years. Given the improved imaging made possible by transrectal ultrasonography, the problem of poor placement has been corrected, and brachytherapy is once again considered a treatment option.[10,11]

Permanent seed implants contain either iodine 125 or palladium 103. The implantation can be performed as an outpatient procedure with spinal anesthesia. Transrectal ultrasonography guidance is used to insert needles through the perineal skin according to a predrilled template, which ensures correct spacing. A string of radioactive seeds is inserted along each needle track. Depending on the size of the prostate, the patient will need 75 to 120 seeds.

Patients should be carefully selected for this type of treatment. They should have low-volume tumours, preferably stage T1c (determined by needle biopsy after a high PSA test result) or T2a, with a Gleason score of less than 7.[10] A matched peripheral dose of 145 Gy is usually prescribed, the rectal wall receiving 100 Gy. The sequelae are acceptable and include acute proctitis (occurring in up to 25% of patients) and urethritis (dysuria, nocturia and increased frequency, which occur in up to 45% of patients and which usually last for about 2 months but can persist for up to 4–6 months). The most common late sequelae have been incontinence (in up to 5% of patients) and urethral stricture (in 12%), but the risk of these problems has been reduced recently by peripheral loading of the implants, which spares the urethra, and by avoidance of transurethral prostate resection after implantation. Prolonged urinary symptoms should be managed conservatively. Late proctitis occurs in only 3% of patients.

Overall outlook for radiotherapy

Both 3-dimensional conformal radiotherapy and brachytherapy offer significant improvements in the ability to deliver a high dose of radiation to the prostate while sparing the radiosensitive adjacent organs. The short- and intermediate-term results for these treatments are promising. For patients with bulkier tumours or higher Gleason scores, distant failure remains a significant problem, and continuing assessment and exploration of combined modes of treatment are needed to address the systemic component of the disease.

Treating hormone-refractory prostate cancer

Hormone-refractory prostate cancer is prostate cancer that continues to progress after initial or sequential hormonal therapies to suppress the production or activity of testicular and adrenal androgens and after withdrawal of the anti-androgen.

Hormonal treatment of prostate cancer can take several forms.[12] In about 70% to 80% of patients with metastatic prostate cancer, the disease responds to primary androgen ablation therapy — orchidectomy or administration of luteininzing hormone-releasing hormone (LHRH) agonist — as indicated by relief of symptoms and a fall in the PSA level. The duration of such response is variable but averages about 1 year. Although the results of a meta-analysis[13] and a recent large US intergroup trial[14] do not suggest any survival benefit from initial combined androgen blockade, the addition of an anti-androgen at the time of disease progression can lead to a transient further response in about 30% of patients.[15] Moreover, withdrawal of the anti-androgen can also lead to a response (in terms of both symptoms and PSA level) in about 20% of patients whose disease responds to initial androgen ablation therapy.[16,17] There are also rare, but well-documented, examples of response after the reintroduction of hormonal agents in patients whose disease progressed after each of the above manoeuvres[15] and whose disease would thus have been considered hormone refractory. Although this tertiary response occurs much too rarely for reintroduction of hormone therapy to be regarded as standard management, it illustrates our limited understanding of the nature of hormonal resistance in prostate cancer.

In parallel with these observations, several recent studies have investigated genetic changes in the androgen receptor in patients with apparent hormone resistance and the influence of such changes on response to hormone manipulation in tissue culture and in animal models. Point mutations in the androgen receptor gene of prostate cancer cells generally lead to nonfunctioning of the receptor and impart resistance to further hormone manipulation.[18,19] Conversely, some tumours may develop amplification of the unmodified androgen receptor gene and may respond to further hormonal manipulation.[20]

The current definition of hormone-refractory prostate cancer will probably be modified on the basis of molecular studies of the androgen receptor gene and other genes that influence its expression. Questions about benefit or harm from continuing or discontinuing LHRH agonists in the face of apparent hormonal resistance will also be addressed at the clinical and molecular levels: an initial trial to address clinical aspects of this question is in progress (I.F.T., unpublished data). In the future, molecular studies of prostate cancer biopsy samples from patients whose disease appears refractory to standard endocrine therapy will be used to identify a subpopulation of patients who might benefit from further hormonal manipulation.

Treatment of symptoms

The main symptoms associated with hormone-refractory prostate cancer are pain from bone metastases and fatigue. Patients with these symptoms require optimal analgesic medication and radiation therapy for painful secondary bone lesions. This type of supportive care is likely to remain the cornerstone of patient management.

There is considerable scope for improvement in pain control and in the aggressive management of the complications of narcotic medication that limit tolerance of such drugs. The routine assessment of pain during each visit to the clinic or office (for example, by the simple means of asking the patient to rate his pain on a scale of 0 to 10) can do much to improve the recognition and treatment of pain and thus to improve patients' quality of life.

Recent randomized controlled trials using validated symptomatic endpoints have shown substantial reductions in pain in patients with hormone-refractory prostate cancer who underwent 1 of 2 treatments:
- administration of strontium 89, which has physicochemical properties similar to those of calcium and is taken up by sclerotic bone, where it provides local irradiation of bone lesions[21–23]
- chemotherapy with mitoxantrone and prednisone.[12,24]

> **KEY POINTS**
> - More information about the nature of hormone-refractory prostate cancer (progression of disease after initial or sequential hormonal therapy and withdrawal of anti-androgen) is likely to come from molecular studies of the androgen receptor gene and other genes that influence its expression.
> - Two treatments have been shown to relieve pain and improve the quality of life of patients with hormone-refractory prostate cancer: strontium 89 for secondary bone lesions and chemotherapy with mitoxantrone and prednisone.
> - Increased understanding of the biology of prostate cancer is leading to investigation of innovative biological strategies, such as suppression of blood vessel proliferation, inhibition of growth factors, stimulation of programmed cell death, cultivation of a patient's own antigen-presenting cells and gene therapy.

^{89}Sr, when given with conventional radiotherapy, decreased bone pain and delayed the onset of pain at new sites when given with conventional radiotherapy, relative to conventional radiotherapy alone.[21,22] Treatment with mitoxantrone (a gentle anticancer drug) and prednisone provided considerably greater and longer-duration pain relief than prednisone alone and delayed the progression of symptoms.[24] The crossover design of the trial prevented assessment of effects on survival. Mitoxantrone is well tolerated, and its use led to improvements in aspects of quality of life other than pain, as well as a greater probability of fall in PSA (a further review of the data has shown that 39% of the patients taking mitoxantrone and prednisone had a 50% or greater decrease in PSA measured on at least 2 occasions, whereas only 16% of patients taking prednisone alone showed this degree of PSA decline; $p = 0.001$). However, reduction in PSA and symptomatic response are imperfectly correlated, and the level of PSA was not at all useful in predicting the survival of patients with hormone-refractory prostate cancer.[24]

Several other anticancer drugs may lead to a decrease in PSA levels and to a decrease in pain (as assessed by physicians) in patients with hormone-refractory prostate cancer. These might provide alternatives to palliation for such patients, or they might add to the effects of mitoxantrone if used in combination with that drug. However, there is no evidence to suggest that any of the current anticancer drugs will have a major impact on survival, and the use of more toxic compounds in elderly men is likely to detract from palliation rather than add to it. Studies of high-dose mitoxantrone or highly emetogenic drugs such as cisplatin seem misguided. Mitoxantrone was chosen for study because it is a drug that is well-tolerated by older people; therefore, it would be appropriate to test other well-tolerated anticancer drugs using similar endpoints to assess palliative benefit.

Another class of drugs, the bisphosphonates, inhibit resorption of bone and have been shown to decrease pain and improve quality of life in patients with other malignant diseases, such as breast cancer and multiple myeloma. Although secondary bone lesions from prostate cancer are largely sclerotic, preliminary evidence from phase II trials indicates that bisphosphonates might convey similar benefit to patients with hormone-refractory prostate cancer.[25] The current National Cancer Institute of Canada randomized double-blind trial for patients with symptomatic hormone-refractory prostate cancer is examining pain and quality of life in patients who receive mitoxantrone and prednisone in combination with either clodronate or placebo.

Novel approaches

Increases in our understanding of the biology of cancer, and of prostate cancer in particular, are leading to trials of strategies involving biological agents (Table 1). Because prostate cancer may progress relatively slowly (although the median survival from time of development of hormone

Table 1: New biological strategies for the treatment of prostate cancer

Strategy	Mechanism
Anti-angiogenesis	Tumour growth depends on new blood vessels. Tumour cells secrete growth factors (e.g., vascular endothelial growth factor) that bind to receptors on endothelial cells to stimulate their proliferation. Some agents interrupt this pathway.
Inhibition of growth-factor receptors on tumour cells	Malignant cells (including those in prostate tumours) depend on stimulating growth factors that bind to specific receptors. Some agents prevent such binding.
Differentiation therapy	Cancer cells may undergo tissue-specific differentiation or proliferation. Some agents stimulate differentiation and inhibit proliferation.
Stimulation of apoptosis	Apoptosis (programmed cell death) occurs after androgen withdrawal in hormone-sensitive prostate cancer. Stimulation of the genes that promote apoptosis (e.g., *bax*) or antisense constructs to genes that inhibit it (e.g., *bcl2*) might cause cell death in hormone-refractory prostate cancer.
Immunologic approaches	Recent advances in our understanding of the molecular complexity of the immune system allow new approaches, including the isolation and cultivation of a patient's own antigen-presenting cells (dendritic cells) followed by reinfusion.
Gene therapy	Various genes can cause death of the cells into which they are introduced, either directly or by stimulating immune mechanisms. The key to this approach is to develop strategies that allow insertion of specific genes into prostate cancer cells. One method is to use viruses that seek cells producing prostate-specific antigen to insert these "suicide" genes.

resistance is only about 1 year), there is an opportunity to evaluate long-term treatments, such as agents to inhibit formation of the new blood vessels required for tumour growth.

The approaches listed in Table 1 are more likely to result in small, gradual advances than in dramatic breakthroughs. These agents, and others as they become available, should be evaluated in translational trials that evaluate tumour reduction or inhibition of growth, as measured by PSA and other markers; reduction of pain and other symptoms and effects on global quality of life; and genetic and cellular changes in the patient's tumour cells, to allow clinical and biological correlation.

Cancer cells are remarkably effective at becoming resistant to almost any therapy. In addition, biological therapies usually exert their greatest effects when tumours are small. Thus, if such approaches are to have an impact on the prevalence of hormone-refractory prostate cancer, they will probably have to be used in combination with hormonal manipulation at relatively early stages of disease to delay or prevent progression to the hormone-refractory state.

References

1. Goldenberg SL, Ramsey EW, Jewett MAS. Prostate cancer: 6. Surgical treatment of localized disease. *CMAJ* 1998;159(10):1265-71. [Chapter 6 in this book.]
2. Corral D, Pisters L, von Eschenbach A. Treatment options for localized prostate cancer following radiation therapy. *Urol Clin North Am* 1996;23(4):677-84.
3. Cespedes DR, Pisters LL, von Eschenbach AC, McGuire EJ. Long-term follow up of incontinence and obstruction after salvage cryosurgical ablation of the prostate: results in 143 patients. *J Urol* 1997;157:237-40.
4. Gelet A, Dubernard JM, Cathignol D, Abdelrahim AF, Pangaud C, Souchon R, et al. Treatment of prostate cancer with transrectal focussed ultrasound: early clinical experience. *Eur Urol* 1996;29:174-83.
5. Gelet A, Dubernard JM, Cathignol D, Blanc E, Souchon R, Pangaud C, et al. Preliminary results of the treatment of 44 patients with localized cancer of the prostate using transrectal focussed ultrasound. *Prog Urol* 1998;8:68-77.
6. Lancaster C, Toi A, Trachtenberg J. Interstitial microwave thermoablation for localized prostate cancer. *Urology* 1999;53(4):828-31.
7. Trachtenberg J, Kucharczyk W, Chen J, Murphy S, Lancaster C, Toi A, et al. Interstitial microwave thermoablation for localized prostate cancer after failed radiation therapy. In: Bodmer W, editor. *New perspectives in prostate cancer.* 2nd ed. Oxford: Isis Medical Media; 1999.
8. Kupelian P, Katcher J, Levin H, Zippe C, Soh J, Macklis R, et al. External beam radiotherapy vs radical prostatectomy for clinical stage T1–T2 prostate cancer: therapeutic implications of stratification by pretreatment PSA levels and biopsy Gleason score. *Cancer J Sci Am* 1994;3(2):78-87.
9. Hanks GE, Lee WR, Hanlon AL, Hunt M, Kaplan E, Epstein BE, et al. Conformal technique dose escalation for prostate cancer: biochemical evidence of improved cancer control with higher doses in patients with pretreatment prostate-specific antigen ≥10 ng/mL. *Int J Radiat Oncol Biol Phys* 1996;35:861-8.

10. Warde P, Catton C, Gospodarowicz MK. Prostate cancer: 7. Radiation therapy for localized disease. *CMAJ* 1998;159(11):1381-8. [Chapter 7 in this book.]
11. Ragde H, Blasko JC, Grimm PD, Kenny GM, Sylvester JE, Hoak DC, et al. Interstitial iodine-125 radiation without adjuvant therapy in the treatment of clinically localized prostate carcinoma. *Cancer* 1997;80:442-53.
12. Gleave ME, Bruchovsky N, Moore MJ, Venner P. Prostate cancer: 9. Treatment of advanced disease. *CMAJ* 1999;160(2):225-32. [Chapter 9 in this book.]
13. Eisenberger M, Crawford ED, McLeod D, Loehrer P, Wilding G, Blumenstein B. A comparison of bilateral orchiectomy with or without flutamide in stage D2 prostate cancer [abstract]. *Proc Am Soc Clin Oncol* 1997;16:2a.
14. Prostate Cancer Trialists' Collaborative Group. Maximum androgen blockade in advanced prostate cancer: an overview of 22 randomised trials with 3283 deaths in 5710 patients. *Lancet* 1995;346:265-9.
15. Dowling AG, Tannock IF. Systemic treatment for prostate cancer. *Cancer Treat Rev* 1998;24:283-301.
16. Scher HI, Zhang ZF, Nanus D, Kelly WK. Hormone and antihormone withdrawal: implications for the management of androgen-independent prostate cancer. *Urology* 1996;47:61-9.
17. Small EJ, Vogelzang NJ. Second-line hormonal therapy for advanced prostate cancer: a shifting paradigm. *J Clin Oncol* 1997;15:382-8.
18. Taplin ME, Bubley GJ, Shuster TD, Frantz ME, Spooner AE, Ogata GK, et al. Mutation of the androgen-receptor gene in metastatic androgen-independent prostate cancer. *N Engl J Med* 1995;332:1393-8.
19. Tilley WD, Buchanan G, Hickey TE, Bentel JM. Mutations in the androgen receptor gene are associated with progression of human prostate cancer to androgen independence. *Clin Cancer Res* 1996;2:277-85.
20. Koivisto P, Kononen J, Palmberg C, Tammela T, Hyytinen E, Isola J, et al. Androgen receptor gene amplification: a possible molecular mechanism for androgen deprivation therapy failure in prostate cancer. *Cancer Res* 1997;57:314-9.
21. Porter AT, McEwan AJ, Powe JE, Reid R, McGowan DG, Lukka H, et al. Results of a randomized phase-III trial to evaluate the efficacy of strontium-89 adjuvant to local field external beam irradiation in the management of endocrine resistant metastatic prostate cancer. *Int J Radiat Oncol Biol Phys* 1993;25:805-13.
22. Quilty PM, Kirk D, Bolger JJ, Dearnaley DP, Lewington VJ, Mason MD, et al. A comparison of the palliative effects of strontium-89 and external beam radiotherapy in metastatic prostate cancer. *Radiother Oncol* 1994;31:33-40.
23. Iscoe NA, Bruera E, Choo RC. Prostate cancer: 10. Palliative care. *CMAJ* 1999;160(3):365-71. [Chapter 10 in this book.]
24. Tannock IF, Osoba D, Stockler MR, Ernst DS, Neville AJ, Moore MJ, et al. Chemotherapy with mitoxantrone plus prednisone or prednisone alone for symptomatic hormone-resistant prostate cancer: a Canadian randomized trial with palliative endpoints. *J Clin Oncol* 1996;14:1756-64.
25. Cresswell SM, English PJ, Hall RR, Roberts JT, Marsh MM. Pain relief and quality-of-life assessment following intravenous and oral clodronate in hormone-escaped metastatic prostate cancer. *Br J Urol* 1995;76:360-5.

12

The economic burden

Steven A. Grover, MD, MPA; Hanna Zowall, MA; Louis Coupal, MSc; Murray D. Krahn, MD, MSc

The economic burden of prostate cancer is substantial and growing. The diagnosis of new cases has been increasing at an exponential rate since 1990, largely as the result of increased use of prostate-specific antigen (PSA) testing for screening.[1] Demographic trends in the next 20 years will exacerbate the effects of changing disease epidemiology by increasing the population of older men at risk for prostate cancer. Statistics Canada projections indicate that the population of men over age 40 will increase from 5.7 million in 1995 to 9 million in 2016, an increase of 57%.[2] New diagnostic and therapeutic procedures — testing for total PSA and free PSA, nerve-sparing radical prostatectomy, cryotherapy, gene therapy and others — continue to be developed and widely used. These will inevitably put additional demands on our health care resources.

Health care needs are unlimited, whereas resources are finite. Public expenditures on health care have to compete with other societal priorities such as education, the environment, defence and infrastructure. Even in relatively wealthy, developed countries, scarcity is the defining characteristic of resource allocation problems. Economic studies are playing an increasing role in helping both clinicians and the institutions that fund and provide health care to evaluate resource allocation challenges in a rational, evidence-based manner.

Defining and estimating the cost of disease

The economic burden of any disease can be defined in terms of the direct and indirect costs incurred by patients and society as a whole. The direct costs reflect the value of goods and services for health care or resources that could have been used for other purposes in the absence of illness.[3] These include the costs of care provided by physicians and other health care professionals, care provided in hospitals and other health care institutions, drugs, laboratory services and research. The indirect costs represent the reduced productivity associated with lost or impaired ability to work because of illness and the loss of economic productivity because of premature death. Thus, we can distinguish between morbidity costs and mortality costs. Indirect costs are more elusive than direct costs, because economic valuation of life in sickness and in health is beset by methodologic and measurement difficulties.

There are 2 main approaches to estimating indirect costs: the human capital method and the willingness-to-pay approach. The first evaluates productivity lost because of disability or premature death, on the basis of lost earnings.[4-7] Conversely, the willingness-to-pay approach considers the amount people are willing to pay to reduce the risk of illness or death.[4-6,8] In most instances, willingness-to-pay estimates are higher than those based on foregone earnings. The human capital approach, although widely used because of the availability of reliable statistics on individual income and earnings, is often criticized because it tends to discriminate against economically disadvantaged people and groups with lower rates of participation in the labour force, such as women, young people, those with disabilities and elderly people.

Direct costs of prostate cancer

Because prostate cancer develops slowly and affects men in the later

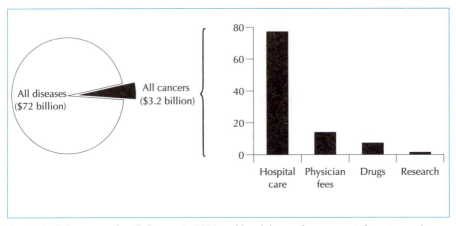

Fig. 1: Total direct costs for all diseases in 1993 and breakdown of cancer costs by category.[3]

stages of their lives, one might expect most prostate cancer costs to be associated with direct health care expenditures (related to detection, initial and follow-up treatments, and treatments of complications due to these interventions) rather than the indirect costs associated with illness and death. According to Health Canada estimates,[3] of the $72 billion in total direct costs for all diseases in 1993, direct costs for all forms of cancer amounted to $3.2 billion, and of this amount, more than three-quarters was spent on hospital care alone; physician fees, drugs and research accounted for much smaller proportions of the total (Fig. 1).

Unfortunately, no Canadian data are available on the direct costs of prostate cancer. However, in the Netherlands, prostate cancer accounted for 5% to 6% of direct health care costs for all cancers in 1988.[9] In Sweden these costs have been estimated at 5.8% of the total costs for all tumours.[10] If a similar percentage is assumed for Canada, the direct costs of treating prostate cancer in this country could be estimated at $193 million. This seems relatively small in relation to other diseases (Table 1).

In Sweden the average cost per patient from diagnosis until death was estimated at $12 400 (in 1985 US dollars).[10] Approximately 25% of total costs for medical care were incurred during the first year after diagnosis. Hospital costs were responsible for the largest share of the total (72%), whereas drugs accounted for approximately 15% of the total. A Norwegian study demonstrated substantial requirements for treatment and care from diagnosis until death, even among patients treated conservatively (i.e., with noncurative intent).[11] For instance, 49% of the patients reported complications requiring admission to hospital, 66% required various prostatic surgical procedures, and 76% needed androgen ablation. Palliative irradiation was given to 16% of the patients, and half received analgesics regularly.

In the United States the cost of treatments for localized prostate cancer was estimated at $10 000 to $20 000 per patient; estimates for treatment of advanced disease ranged from $30 000 to $100 000 per patient.[12] In an analysis of data from a health maintenance organization, the costs of initial care — within the first 6 months after

Table 1: Direct costs of selected diseases in Canada, 1993*

Disease or condition	Estimated cost, $ (and %)
Prostate cancer†	193 (0.3)
Breast and female genital cancers	329 (0.5)
All cancers	3 222 (4.5)
Birth defects	305 (0.4)
Diabetes	577 (0.8)
Infectious and parasitic diseases	787 (1.1)
Stroke	1 445 (2.0)
Coronary artery disease	2 075 (2.9)
All diseases	71 743 (100)

*Source: Moore and associates.[3]
†Estimate is based on the assumption that 6% of direct costs for all cancers is attributable to prostate cancer.

> **KEY POINTS**
> - The economic burden of prostate cancer is substantial, and, as the so-called baby boomers enter their 50s and 60s, the population of men at risk for prostate cancer will increase rapidly.
> - The economic burden of any disease is the sum of the direct and indirect costs to both patients and society.
> - Direct costs are costs of care provided by physicians and other health care professionals, care provided in hospitals and other health care institutions, drugs, laboratory services and research.
> - Indirect costs represent the reduced productivity associated with inability to work because of illness and the loss of economic productivity because of premature death.

diagnosis — were estimated at $1500 per month (in 1992 US dollars) among men 65 to 79 years old.[13] Surprisingly, the costs of initial care did not vary much with stage of disease or coexisting conditions but did decrease with age to $1100 per month for those over 80. The mean cost of continuing care was estimated at $500 per month. The cost of terminal care — care during the last 6 months of life — increased substantially, to over $2700 per month, depending on the stage of the cancer, the patient's age and the extent of coexisting conditions. In a Canadian study of patients with end-stage prostate cancer, the monthly cost of total medical care for those treated with strontium 89 (excluding the initial costs of the strontium) was estimated at $1404 per patient (in 1989 Canadian dollars).[14]

Although these studies provide estimates of the direct costs of prostate cancer, the data may be rapidly becoming dated. Patterns of care for prostate cancer changed dramatically between 1984 and 1990.[15] Among patients in whom prostate cancer had been newly diagnosed, use of PSA testing increased from 5% in 1984 to 66% in 1990, and the use of transrectal ultrasonography rose from less than 1% to 20% during this time. Use of computed tomography and magnetic resonance imaging also increased in this patient group, from 20% to 34% and from 2% to 5% respectively, between 1984 and 1990. Overall, the use of diagnostic tests increased, whereas the proportion of abnormal findings did not. Use of radical prostatectomy as the initial treatment increased from 9% of patients in 1984 to 24% in 1990; the use of radiation therapy remained unchanged. On the other hand, the proportion of patients in whom cancer had been newly diagnosed and who were receiving no initial treatment declined from 36% in 1984 to 29% in 1990.[15,16] These trends have contributed significantly to the increases in the costs of prostate cancer treatment.

In Canada there is little information on the changing patterns of prostate cancer care compatible with the data from the United States. However, some fragmented provincial data are available. For example, in

Saskatchewan the use of PSA testing increased from 100 tests per month in 1990 to more than 4000 in 1994.[17] Concordantly, the number of prostate biopsies increased substantially over the same period. However, prostate cancer was diagnosed in only 35% of the men with abnormal PSA levels (greater than 10 ng/mL) who underwent biopsy. The use of PSA testing also increased exponentially elsewhere in Canada between 1988 and 1996 (e.g., in Ontario[18] and British Columbia [Martin Townson, Information and Analysis Branch, BC Ministry of Health and Ministry Responsible for Seniors, Victoria: personal communication, 1998]).

In Ontario the annual number of radical prostatectomy procedures among men over 49 years of age increased from 239 in 1989 to 1081 in 1994.[19] The largest increases were among men 50–64 years of age. The hospital admission costs associated with radical prostatectomy and orchidectomy in Canada have recently been calculated (by S.A.G. and colleagues, using methodology of the Canadian Institute for Health Information[20]) (Table 2). The physician fees associated with these hospital admissions have been estimated on the basis of the mean of the Ontario and Quebec reimbursement schedules.[22–24] The hospital cost of radical prostatectomy has been estimated at $6825 and the associated physician fees at $1442. Accordingly, the increase in the number of radical prostatectomies performed between 1989 and 1994 in Ontario alone might have resulted in $7 million in additional expenditures.

Prostate cancer is a disease that evolves

Table 2: Mean hospital costs and length of stay for patients with prostate cancer*

Type of hospital care	Mean length of stay, d	Costs, $ Hospital charges	Costs, $ Physician fees	Costs, $ Total
Initial therapy				
Radical prostatectomy	7.7	6 825	1 442	8 267
External-beam radiotherapy†	—‡	4 860	400	5 260
Endocrine therapy (orchidectomy)	1.0	1 105	585	1 689
Treatment of complications after initial therapy				
Bowel or rectal surgical injury	12.2	10 030	758	10 788
Urethral stricture	1.0	512	329	842
Implantation of urinary sphincter	1.0	4 649	530	5 179
Penile prosthesis	1.0	4 649	391	5 041
Cardiopulmonary complications	7.4	5 565	376	5 941
Vascular complications	7.4	4 079	317	4 396
Radiation-related complications				
Cystitis	5.4	3 098	246	3 345
Hematuria	3.3	2 018	178	2 196
Proctitis or rectal stricture	1.0	695	271	966
Diarrhea	4.0	2 627	200	2 827

*Source: S.A. Grover and colleagues (unpublished data), except as noted otherwise. Costs are in 1996 Canadian dollars. Some rows do not sum to total given because of rounding.
†Source: reference 21.
‡This type of therapy is provided mainly on an outpatient basis in hospital clinics.

> **KEY POINTS**
> - Cost-of-illness studies allow us to identify general categories of heavy resource use.
> - Cost-effectiveness studies can guide health care decisions by estimating the relation between resource use and the health outputs of a given program; they provide an assessment of "value for money."
> - As the economic burden of prostate cancer rises over the coming decades, cost-of-illness estimates will allow us to forecast future health care expenditures, and cost-effectiveness studies will show us whether increased spending on early screening, staging, and curative or palliative interventions can be offset by either savings or health benefits.

over a relatively long period. Hence, the costs of follow-up treatment may be particularly important. For example, in the United States the 5-year cumulative incidence of additional cancer treatment after radical prostatectomy was recently estimated at 35%.[25] Even for patients with pathologically organ-confined cancer, the 5-year cumulative incidence was 24%. Thus, the costs of follow-up treatments, even for cancers that are clinically insignificant at diagnosis, may be substantial.

The costs of treating complications arising from initial treatment could be significant as well. For example, serious cardiopulmonary complications requiring admission to hospital occurred in 7% of men aged 75–79 years after radical prostatectomy.[26] These morbidity rates increased to 10% for those aged 80 and over. In a review of treatments for localized prostate cancer,[27] average mortality rates due to radical prostatectomy and external-beam radiation therapy were estimated at 1.1% and 0.2% respectively. The probability of becoming incontinent after surgery or radiation was estimated at 27% and 6% respectively. The prevalence of complete incontinence was estimated at 7% for patients who had undergone surgery and over 1% for those who had undergone radiation therapy. Erectile dysfunction was estimated to occur in 85% of patients who had undergone surgery and 41% of those who had undergone radiation therapy. Canadian hospital admission costs for treating complications arising from the initial surgery or radiation therapy have also been calculated (Table 2). Clearly these costs are important.

There are at present no Canadian estimates of the total expenditures on drugs associated with the treatment of prostate cancer. However, of the total $234 million spent on drug expenditures for all forms of cancer in 1993, 26% ($60 million) was spent on breast and female genital cancers.[3] Given the comparable prevalence of prostate cancer and the common use of androgen blockade, one might expect substantial drug costs for prostate cancer as well. Moreover, these costs are rising and will continue to increase with greater numbers of patients.

For example, according to data from the Ontario Drug Benefit (ODB)

Program,[28] total drug expenditures for prostate cancer treatments among men over 64 years of age increased from $0.2 million in 1985 to over $15 million in 1992 (a 70-fold increase). Over the same period, the ODB Program costs for all drugs increased from $212 million to $646 million (a 3-fold increase).[29] The number of cases of prostate cancer diagnosed annually increased from 2795 in 1985 to 8376 in 1992, and the estimated annual drug cost per cancer patient increased from $77 in 1985 to $1838 in 1992 (a 24-fold increase).[28] At the same time, the ODB Program costs per patient for all drugs increased from $221 to $530 (a 2-fold increase).[29]

Although some of the cost increase for prostate cancer drugs was a result of more cases and increased charges for individual drugs, the majority was due to the use of new drugs. In 1985 most patients were treated with the relatively inexpensive conjugated estrogen diethylstilbestrol, which had become less popular by 1990 because of its cardiovascular side effects.

Indirect costs of prostate cancer

At present there are few data on which to base estimates of the costs of disability and premature death caused by prostate cancer in Canada. For all forms of cancer, these costs were calculated at $9.8 billion in 1993.[3] More than $8.8 billion (90%) of this amount was due to the indirect costs associated with premature death. Prostate cancer is responsible for 3.8% of all potential years of life lost.[30] One might, therefore, be tempted to estimate the indirect costs of prostate cancer due to premature death at $334 million in terms of lost productivity, but such a calculation would be crude at best.[31]

Productivity losses have been calculated according to the human capital approach used by Health Canada;[3] this calculation incorporates the value of labour income lost and the replacement value of unpaid work. Most prostate cancer occurs in men aged 70 years and over. Only 15% of Canadians at age 70 are active in the labour force; this proportion drops to 10% at age 75 and to 7% at age 80.[32] At these ages most income is derived from government transfers (public pensions) and accumulated private funds (private pensions and investments). Therefore, the indirect costs of prostate cancer due to premature death estimated by the human capital method may well be less than the $334 million mentioned above. Unfortunately, there are no reported analyses specifically calculating the indirect costs of prostate cancer.

Cost of illness and cost-effectiveness

Why is it important to know the economic burden associated with a given disease? How is this information useful and to whom?

First, cost-of-illness studies allow us to identify, in a broad sense, categories of heavy resource use. They also identify stakeholders in health policy decisions (e.g., pharmaceutical companies and provincial ministries of health) and the relative size of their stakes. Perhaps the most useful role is to facilitate planning for future health care expenditures. It is worth noting, however, that some economists view cost-of-illness studies with suspicion, as they are often used by various interest groups to increase awareness of a specific intervention or disease.[33–35]

What cost-of-illness studies cannot do is show whether more resources should be devoted to the particular health care intervention or the trade-offs involved in choosing between interventions. Simply revealing that prostate cancer costs X dollars is insufficient to indicate whether we should be spending more on prostate cancer research or on new and exciting treatment Y. Such decisions require cost-effectiveness analyses or economic evaluation.

Economic evaluation helps guide decision-making by outlining the relation between resource consumption and the health outputs of a given program; it provides an assessment of "value for money" or the economic efficiency of an intervention, given limited resources.[36] Cost-effectiveness studies ask the following questions: What are the alternatives to treatment Y? How effective are they? How much do they cost? If Y is more effective, is the gain in effectiveness worth the additional cost? Cost-effectiveness studies never provide a definitive answer to these questions, because they inevitably involve questions of values and ethics. However, they do provide a framework to guide decision-making and a starting point for discussion.

Cost-effectiveness studies

Within the last 10 years, an increasing number of studies evaluating the cost-effectiveness of prostate cancer screening, diagnosis and treatment modalities have been published. For example, at least 6 studies have evaluated the role of PSA screening.[21,37–41] All of the studies that measured costs suggested that net costs would increase as a result of screening. Four of the 6 suggested that the harmful consequences of screening might offset the potential health benefits associated with early detection.[21,37,38,41] Two studies suggested that PSA screening might be "cost effective" or economically attractive.[39,40] The heterogeneity of these results is accounted for by differences in methods, lack of high-quality data describing costs and the quality-of-life effects of screening, and, in particular, the lack of data from randomized controlled trials characterizing the effects of screening or treatment on death from cancer. Until such data are published, the cost-effectiveness of PSA screening will be highly speculative.

In addition to research on screening, studies are now being

published that evaluate the cost-effectiveness of the entire diagnostic and treatment cascade. Such studies consider the role of second opinion pathological review,[42] less invasive[43] or less expensive[44,45] staging strategies, early discharge after radical prostatectomy,[46] the use of flutamide[47,48] and the use of palliative chemotherapy for end-stage disease.[49]

Future economic trends

Health care expenditures on prostate cancer are likely to rise in the near future. Even if incidence rates were to remain at their present level, the aging of the population will increase the prevalence of prostate cancer over the next 20 years. Cost-of-illness studies will help to forecast future health care expenditures. Cost-effectiveness studies will determine whether increased spending on early screening, staging, and curative or palliative interventions can be offset by either cost savings or sufficient health benefit (e.g., cancers cured, lives saved or painful metastatic disease prevented) to warrant additional expenditures. To answer these questions, all relevant costs must be accounted for and the clinical evidence of the effectiveness of various prostate cancer treatments must be demonstrated.

Major gaps in scientific knowledge remain as barriers to good economic analyses. The largest of these is the absence of results of randomized controlled trials evaluating the efficacy of alternative screening, staging and treatment interventions. Such trials are under way in the United States and Europe and are planned for Canada. In addition, quality-of-life effects of treatment and screening are not well understood, although evidence is slowly accumulating. Little is known about the utilization patterns of health care services by Canadian urologists and other physicians in the treatment of prostate cancer. Finally, information on outcomes according to age, stage and grade of cancer, and treatment modalities, although difficult to collect, will prove essential in projecting future health care requirements. Better-quality data will put future cost-of-illness studies and, in particular, cost-effectiveness analyses, on a much firmer foundation.

References

1. Levy IG, Iscoe NA, Klotz LH. Prostate cancer: 1. The descriptive epidemiology in Canada. *CMAJ* 1998;159(5):509-13. [Chapter 1 in this book.]
2. *Population projections for Canada, provinces and territories 1993–2016.* Ottawa: Statistics Canada; 1993. Cat no. 91-520.
3. Moore R, Mao Y, Zhang J, Clarke K. *Economic burden of illness in Canada, 1993.* Ottawa: Health Canada; 1997.

4. Cooper BS, Rice DP. The economic costs of illness revisited. *Soc Secur Bull* 1976;39:21-36.
5. Hodgson TA. The state of the art of cost-of-illness estimates. *Adv Health Econ Health Serv Res* 1983;4:129-64.
6. Robinson JC. Philosophical origins of the economic valuation of life. *Millbank Q* 1986;64:133-55.
7. Rice DP. Estimating the cost of illness. Washington: US Department of Health, Education and Welfare; 1966. Public Health Service, Health Economics Series 6.
8. O'Brien B, Viramontes JL. Willingness to pay: a valid and reliable measure of health state preference. *Med Decis Making* 1994;14:289-97.
9. Koopmanschap MA, Roijen LV, Bonneux L, Barendregt JJ. Current and future costs of cancer. *Eur J Cancer* 1994;30A:60-5.
10. Carlsson P, Hjertberg H, Jönsson B, Barenhorst E. The cost of prostatic cancer in a defined population. *Scand J Urol Nephrol* 1989;23:93-6.
11. Otnes B, Harvei S, Fossa SD. The burden of prostate cancer from diagnosis until death. *Br J Urol* 1995;76:587-94.
12. Denmeade SR, Isaacs JT. Prostate cancer: Where are we and where are we going? *Br J Urol* 1997;79(Suppl 1):2-7.
13. Taplin SH, Barlow W, Urban N, Mandelson MT, Timlin DJ, Ichikawa L, et al. Stage, age, comorbidity, and direct cost of colon, prostate, and breast cancer care. *J Natl Cancer Inst* 1995;87:417-26.
14. McEwan AJB, Amyotte GA, McGowan DG, MacGillivray JA, Porter AT. A retrospective analysis of the cost effectiveness of treatment with Metastron (^{89}Sr-chloride) in patients with prostate cancer metastatic to bone. *Nucl Med Commun* 1994;15:499-504.
15. Jones GW, Mettlin C, Murphy GP. Patterns of care for carcinoma of the prostate gland: results of a national survey of 1984 and 1990. *J Am Coll Surg* 1995;180:545-54.
16. Mettlin C, Jones GW, Murphy GP. Trends in prostate cancer care in the United States, 1974-1990: observations from the patient care evaluation studies of the American College of Surgeons Commission on Cancer. *CA Cancer J Clin* 1993;43:83-91.
17. *The PSA test in early detection of prostate cancer.* Saskatoon: Health Services Utilization and Research Commission; 1995.
18. Bunting PS, Miyazaki JH, Goel V. Laboratory survey of prostate-specific antigen testing in Ontario. *Clin Biochem* 1998;31:47-9.
19. Variations in selected surgical procedures and medical diagnoses by year and region. In: Goel V, Williams JI, Anderson GM, Blackstien-Hirsch P, Fooks C, Naylor CD, editors. *Patterns of health care in Ontario: the ICES practice atlas.* 2nd ed. Ottawa: Canadian Medical Association; 1996. p. 51-146.
20. *Resource intensity weights: summary of methodology, 1996/97.* Ottawa: Canadian Institute for Health Information; 1996.
21. *Screening for cancer of the prostate: an evaluation of benefits, unwanted health effects and costs.* Montreal: Conseil d'évaluation des technologies de la santé du Québec; 1995.
22. *Manuel des médecins omnipraticiens.* Quebec City: Régie de l'assurance-maladie du Québec; 1996.
23. *Manuel des médecins spécialistes.* Quebec City: Régie de l'assurance-maladie du Québec; 1996.
24. *Schedule of benefits: physician services, 1992.* Toronto: Ontario Ministry of Health; 1992.
25. Lu-Yao GL, Potosky AL, Albertsen PC, Wasson JH, Barry MJ, Wennberg JE. Follow-up prostate cancer treatments after radical prostatectomy: a population-based study. *J*

Natl Cancer Inst 1996;88:166-73.
26. Lu-Yao GL, McLerran D, Wasson J, Wennberg JE. An assessment of radical prostatectomy: time trends, geographic variation, and outcomes. *JAMA* 1993;269:2633-6.
27. Wasson JH, Cushman CC, Bruskewitz RC, Littenberg B, Mulley AG Jr, Wennberg JE. A structured literature review of treatment for localized prostate cancer [published erratum appears in *Arch Fam Med* 1993;2:1030]. *Arch Fam Med* 1993;2:487-93.
28. To T, Iscoe N, Klotz L, Naylor CD. Orchiectomy and hormonal therapy of prostate cancer. *Can J Urol* 1995;2:109-15.
29. Anderson GM. An overview of the use of acute care hospitals, physician and diagnostic services and prescription drugs. In: Naylor CD, Anderson GM, Goel V, editors. *Patterns of health care in Ontario: the ICES practice atlas.* 1st ed. Ottawa: Canadian Medical Association; 1994. p. 21-45.
30. National Cancer Institute of Canada: *Canadian cancer statistics 1997.* Toronto: The Institute; 1997.
31. Morrison HI, MacNeill IB, Miller D, Levy I, Xie L, Mao Y. The impending Canadian prostate cancer epidemic. *Can J Public Health* 1995;86:274-8.
32. Norland JA. *Focus on Canada: profile of Canada's seniors.* Ottawa: Statistics Canada; 1994. Cat no. 96-312E.
33. Drummond MF. Cost-of-illness studies: A major headache? *Pharmacol Econ* 1992;2:1-4.
34. Shiell A, Gerrard K, Donaldson C. Cost of illness studies: An aid to decision-making? *Health Policy* 1987;8:317-23.
35. Hodgson TA. Cost of illness studies: No aid to decision-making? *Health Policy* 1989;11:57-60.
36. Gold MR, Russell LB, Siegel JE, Weinstein MC, editors. *Cost-effectiveness in health and medicine.* Oxford: Oxford University Press; 1996.
37. Krahn MD, Mahoney JE, Eckman MH, Trachtenberg J, Pauker SG, Detsky AS. Screening for prostate cancer: a decision analytic view. *JAMA* 1994;272:781-6.
38. Optenberg SA, Thompson IM. Economics of screening for carcinoma of the prostate. *Urol Clin North Am* 1990;17:719-37.
39. Littrup PJ, Goodman AC, Mettlin CJ. The benefit and cost of prostate cancer early detection. *CA Cancer J Clin* 1993;43:134-49.
40. Coley CM, Barry MJ, Fleming C, Fahs MC, Mulley AG. Early detection of prostate cancer. Part II: Estimating the risks, benefits, and costs. *Ann Intern Med* 1997;126:468-79.
41. Cantor SB, Spann SJ, Volk RJ, Cardenas MP, Warren MM. Prostate cancer screening: a decision analysis. *J Fam Pract* 1995;41:33-41.
42. Epstein JI, Walsh PC, Sanfilippo F. Clinical and cost impact of second-opinion pathology: review of prostate biopsies prior to radical prostatectomy. *Am J Surg Pathol* 1996;20:851-7.
43. Perrotti M, Gentle DL, Barada JH, Wilbur HJ, Kaufman RPJ. Mini-laparotomy pelvic lymph node dissection minimizes morbidity, hospitalization and cost of pelvic lymph node dissection. *J Urol* 1996;155:986-8.
44. Forman HP, Fox LA, Glazer HS, McClennan BL, Anderson DC, Sagel SS. Chest radiography inpatients with early stage prostatic carcinoma. Effect on treatment planning and cost analysis. *Chest* 1994;106:1036-41.
45. Forman HP, Heiken JP, Brink JA, Glazer HS, Fox LA, McClennan BL. CT screening for comorbid disease in patients with prostatic carcinoma: Is it cost-effective? *Am J Roentgenol* 1994;162:1125-8.

46. Licht MR, Klein EA. Early hospital discharge after radical retropubic prostatectomy: impact on cost and complication rate. *Urology* 1994;44:700-4.
47. Hillner BE, McLeod DG, Crawford ED, Bennett CL. Estimating the cost effectiveness of total androgen blockade with flutamide in M1 prostate cancer. *Urology* 1995;45(4):633-40.
48. Bennett CL, Matchar D, McCrory D, McLeod DG, Crawford ED, Hillner BE. Cost-effective models for flutamide for prostate carcinoma patients. Are they helpful to policy makers? *Cancer* 1996;77:1854-61.
49. Bloomfield DJ, Krahn MD, Neogi T, Panzarella T, Smith TJ, Warde P, et al. Economic evaluation of chemotherapy with mitoxantrone plus prednisone for symptomatic hormone-resistant prostate cancer: based on a Canadian randomized trial with palliative end points. *J Clin Oncol* 1998;16:2272-9.

We thank our research assistants Daniel Roth and Annie Bérubé.

13

The view from the other side of the examining table

Ross E. Gray, PhD; Al Philbrook, BA, BLA

Only in the last decade has it been acknowledged broadly that patients need to be involved in planning for and implementing their own health care. The inclusion in this book of a chapter written from the patient's perspective is a welcome extension of this long-overdue trend toward meaningful patient participation.[1,2]

In February 1997 a National Prostate Cancer Forum, with representation from the academic community, health care professionals, administrators and patients, made recommendations to both policy-makers and researchers. The inclusion of patients in this forum added to the richness of the discussions and increased the credibility of the recommendations. Some of the reflections on patient perspectives that we present here are based on experiences from the forum. Another source of information is a 1997 national survey of Canadian men with prostate cancer.[3] We have also drawn on our personal and professional experience in interacting with men who have this disease.

Men with prostate cancer speak with many voices; therefore, it is impossible to present an overall patient perspective. In addition, the men who are more able or willing to voice their opinions or respond to surveys may not always be representative of the larger population of patients with prostate cancer. Finally, not all men are interested in participating in decisions about their own treatment or discussions about the health care system. Despite these issues, we still think there is general agreement among men with prostate cancer about a number of topics, and many of these points of agreement have implications for research.

Patience is a luxury of the well

Michael Milken, who himself has prostate cancer, has argued that the medical and scientific establishment in North America should approach cancer research with more urgency.[4] A wealthy man, he has helped to establish funding for prostate cancer research in the United States. Milken is typical of patients with prostate cancer. They want results. They don't want progress to be held up by inefficient bureaucracies or interdisciplinary politicking. Although they recognize the need for proper scientific investigation of new treatments, they do not want such investigations to drag on interminably when it is clear to all involved that clinical benefits are available.

Canadian patients find it infuriating when promising new treatments are withheld in this country, are accessible only through clinical trials or are offered only at selected facilities. For example, over the past few years, many Canadian prostate cancer patients would have preferred the most recent radiotherapy techniques (e.g., 3-dimensional conformal radiotherapy) as their treatment of choice. However, they had to either travel to the US or choose another treatment that was covered by Canadian health insurance. Could these treatments have been made accessible more quickly? Even if it is impossible to make changes at the pace patients would like, why not try?

We recognize that scientists and health care professionals often share patients' frustration with the slow pace of change. For example, the chapter in this book by Meyer and Fradet[5] describes the terrible scientific impasse we've reached regarding the usefulness of screening for prostate cancer with the prostate-specific antigen (PSA) test. Their recommendation to move forward on the basis of existing evidence, rather than waiting for evidence that may arrive late or not at all, is the kind of reasoning that resonates with patients. Similarly, Gallagher and Fleshner[6] acknowledge that there is as yet no firm evidence to support wide-scale primary prevention trials related to prostate cancer. But they also argue that there *is* enough evidence about the likely benefit of a number of lifestyle interventions to warrant discussing them with patients. Most patients would rather be told that there is something they can do that *might* help prevent the disease or its recurrence than hear that there is insufficient evidence to support any action. Scientists may be able to wait for the final word. Patients can't afford to.

Men need to be educated about the benefits of PSA screening

With reference to screening, we acknowledge the differences in terminology referred to by Meyer and Fradet,[5] and, like them, we assume that screening means "the examination of asymptomatic people in order to classify them as likely, or unlikely, to have the disease that is the object of screening."[7]

Although there are debates about the benefits of PSA screening within the larger health care system, there is little debate on this subject among men with prostate cancer. Many prostate cancer patients feel that their disease might have been cured or that they might have a longer life expectancy if testing had been done earlier. Most feel adamantly that PSA testing should be readily accessible to all men. A core issue is that men believe that they themselves, rather than physicians or health care bureaucrats, should be making decisions about their health care, such as the decision to undergo screening. This sentiment is reflected in a broadly supported recommendation from the national forum, that Canadian men be made aware of the benefits and risks of PSA testing *so that they can make their own informed decisions*.[8] Men with prostate cancer strongly encourage physicians to follow this recommendation.

> **KEY POINTS**
> - Patients can't wait for the final proof — they would rather be told that there is something they can do that *might* help prevent the disease or its recurrence than hear that there is insufficient evidence to support any action.
> - In the midst of the debate over screening for prostate-specific antigen, many believe that men should be making their own informed decisions about their health.
> - Patients want to receive information that is even-handed and acknowledges the potential benefits (and negative consequences) of all possible interventions.
> - Most cancer patients do not get as much information as they would like; printed materials and decision-making aids are helping, but much more could be done.

Communicating information is critical

The importance of information and communication for men with prostate cancer was evident in the findings of the national survey.[3] All types of information was rated as important, and disease and treatment-related information were rated as most important. Even though most of the respondents were satisfied overall with the information they had received and the way in which it had been communicated, there still appeared to be room for improvement. For example, in the domain of supportive care, men's satisfaction was relatively low, which raises questions about how they might better gain access to this type of information. Another important finding was the evidence that many men did not comprehend the information that had been conveyed to them. For example, most respondents said that they had been informed about the stage of their disease and that the staging classification system had been explained to them. Yet most were unable to specify disease stage, typically confusing many different aspects of the medical information that had been communicated to them.

Patients appreciate receiving information that is balanced and that acknowledges the potential benefits (and negative consequences) of all possible interventions. The chapters in this book that discuss various interventions indicate how health care professionals can put forward the merits of a particular approach while respecting other approaches and the central value of patient choice.

Because of the considerable controversy surrounding prostate cancer screening, testing and treatment, it is especially critical that health care professionals adopt a comprehensive approach in communicating information about choices. Although not all men want such information, many of those who are reluctant to ask questions nevertheless do want to understand their medical situation. All evidence suggests that most cancer patients do not get as much information as they would like.[9,10] Development of printed materials and decision-making aids is helping to address this issue for men with prostate cancer, but much more could be done.

In their chapter on palliative care for men with prostate cancer, Iscoe and colleagues[11] discuss the importance of giving patients evidence-based evaluations of experimental and complementary or alternative therapies. We agree that physicians should be balanced in discussing any unproven therapy, whether it's a new chemotherapy drug or a herb from the Amazon. We also agree that it is helpful if they can provide detailed information about what is known about the effects of nonstandard treatments. In one recent study of cancer patients[12] many advocated better access to information about complementary or alternative approaches through their physicians.

Many patients are looking for more than just facts and figures when they raise the possibility of other treatment approaches. Indeed, we believe that most men who pursue complementary approaches know that there is little or no scientific evidence supporting the therapies and that positive benefit may be a long shot. However, they would like their physicians to take their interest in complementary approaches seriously, engage in discussion and be supportive of treatment choices that have little potential for harm. Values other than anticancer effect, such as the patient's religious and cultural beliefs and social and psychological needs, should be included when complementary options are considered. These factors can have every bit as much legitimacy as data from a clinical trial in terms of justifying a decision to try an unconventional approach.

Quality of life cannot be neglected

Around the time of diagnosis, considerations of survival are typically paramount for men with prostate cancer. For those who do well with treatment and have few long-term consequences, there may not be many quality-of-life concerns. Nevertheless, many men experience continuing consequences of illness and treatment, and in cases of recurrent or metastatic disease, quality-of-life concerns become primary.

One of us recently heard a prostate cancer patient tell about his humiliating experience in trying to arrange for a vacuum pump to help him continue an active sex life. He was initially discouraged from investigating this option by his primary care physician, who apparently assumed that sexuality should cease to be of concern after a certain age. Then, when he obtained the device, he had difficulty understanding how it worked and was embarrassed to ask for help. Later, the device broke and he had lengthy negotiations with the manufacturer about getting it fixed.

> **KEY POINTS**
> - For men who experience the ongoing consequences of illness and treatment, quality-of life concerns become primary.
> - Discussion of sensitive issues, such as erectile dysfunction, is often uncomfortable for both patients and busy health care professionals; self-help and support groups can be a good source of helpful information.
> - Cancer patients want someone to spend time with them, to help explain the issues, to answer their questions and to help them navigate through the system.
> - Continuity of care — another often-expressed need of prostate cancer patients — can often best be provided by the primary care physician.
> - Although most men are more concerned with gathering information than expressing feelings, many benefit from and enjoy the supportive components of self-help groups.

This story reveals some of the struggles that men often face, yet is silent about other struggles that are inevitable for couples working out a new approach to lovemaking.

Half of the respondents in the national survey[3] identified sexual function as a problem. In response to an open-ended question about the impact of the disease and treatment on their quality of life, many of the men described the distress they experienced. Of those who identified sexuality as a problem, only 20% reported having received adequate help. Although some of this inaction may have been due to the patients' choosing not to investigate treatment options, systemic barriers probably contributed (e.g., the discomfort of health care professionals in discussing sexual dysfunction and the lack of time in busy clinical practices to deal with sensitive issues). With the promising new treatments now available for erectile dysfunction, as discussed by Hassouna and Heaton,[13] it will become even more important for health care professionals to engage their patients in discussions of the options.

Another quality-of-life issue for some men with prostate cancer is urinary incontinence, a problem well elucidated by Hassouna and Heaton.[13] In the national survey,[3] a minority of men who reported incontinence felt that they had received adequate help. Interestingly, details such as what types of pads work best are often learned from other patients in support and self-help groups. Encouragement from physicians to attend a prostate cancer support group will increase the likelihood of patients participating and, consequently, their access to helpful information.

We commend the focus in this book on the treatment of metastatic disease and the management of medical issues related to advanced disease and dying.[11,14] There is a pressing need for additional research in this area.

Sensitive treatment and care must be a priority

In addition to the topics already covered in this book, a number of psychosocial dimensions of care need attention. There are no easy prescriptions for what constitutes a "sensitive" approach for physician–patient encounters in the context of prostate cancer. At a basic level, the physician should establish a welcoming physical environment, choose a receptionist who puts people at ease, provide relevant reading materials and include the spouse in discussions and deliberations.

One of the concerns we have heard most often is the feeling of being alone in navigating the steps of diagnosis, treatment and follow-up care. It is so easy for older men to get lost in the system, to miss making the necessary appointments, to get confused about what steps to take next, to feel that there is no single professional who has the time or the inclination to help chart his course. The phrase "falling through the cracks" has been used to describe the situation of many patients. In a recent study of cancer patients,[15] a substantial number of respondents indicated a desire to have access to someone who might be able to spend more time with them than their cancer specialist, someone who could help explain the issues, answer their questions and help them to navigate through the system. For some, this role was already being played by their primary care physician or a nurse at a cancer treatment centre.

Another need commonly expressed by cancer patients is continuity of care. Ensuring such continuity should perhaps be the role of the primary care physician, but this role has not always been adequately fulfilled. Too often, it has been left to specialists or the staff of cancer treatment centres to respond to patients' needs. In the national survey[3] only 51% of respondents agreed that their primary care physician was part of their treatment team. Responses to open-ended questions pointed to men's desire for contact with primary care physicians who would be willing to help them negotiate the sometimes-daunting path of their illness. The need for extra time for discussion is especially critical after the initial diagnosis, when men have so many options to consider. Support groups may play a role by giving men opportunities to hear about others' experiences with various treatments. Men who live in rural areas may especially need support from their primary care physicians because of limited access to both cancer specialists and self-help groups.

Men need independence but also appreciate help

Most men express little interest in receiving psychological support or talking about problems.[3] They want to be treated as competent adults, not as sick, vulnerable people. They are more concerned with proactive gathering of information than with expressing feelings. These preferences must be considered when interacting with men with prostate cancer. Yet a recent study of men in prostate cancer self-help groups reported that many benefited from and enjoyed the supportive components of the groups, despite the fact that they had initially attended just to obtain information.[16] This suggests that both components need to be taken seriously by health care professionals. The desire to remain independent should be recognized and facilitated, but efforts should be made to accommodate the need for sharing, whether through support and self-help groups, family discussions or formal counselling.

Conclusion

Men with prostate cancer typically share a sense of urgency about their individual and collective health. They want their sons and grandsons to be able to avoid what has happened to them, and they want researchers to search for the necessary answers. Men also want to be treated well and with respect. They want health care professionals to spend time explaining complex options, and they want to know that there is at least one professional who can be counted on to help them pull all the threads together. They want help in sustaining the best possible quality for their lives.

Many men with prostate cancer are grateful for the assistance that primary care physicians have provided. But others would have liked more assistance, more time. On their behalf, we ask you to consider what is possible.

References

1. Gray RE. Persons with cancer speak out: reflections on an important trend in Canadian health care. *J Palliat Care* 1992;8(4):30-7.
2. Charles C, DeMaio S. Lay participation in health care decision making: a conceptual framework. *J Health Polit Policy Law* 1993;18:881-904.
3. Gray RE, Klotz LH, Iscoe NA, Fitch MI, Franssen E, Johnson BJ, et al. Results of a survey of Canadian men with prostate cancer. *Can J Urol* 1997;4:359-65.

4. Kasindorf JR. What to make of Mike. *Fortune* 1996;134(6):86-9.
5. Meyer F, Fradet Y. Prostate cancer: 4. Screening. *CMAJ* 1998;159(8):968-72. [Chapter 4 in this book.]
6. Gallagher RP, Fleshner N. Prostate cancer: 3. Individual risk factors. *CMAJ* 1998;159(7):807-13. [Chapter 3 in this book.]
7. Morrison AS. *Screening in chronic disease.* New York: Oxford University Press; 1985. p. 3.
8. Phillips R, editor. *Call for action on prostate cancer. Report and recommendations from the 1997 National Prostate Cancer Forum.* Toronto: Canadian Cancer Society; 1997.
9. Houts PS, Yasko JM, Harvey HA, Kahn SB, Hartz AJ, Hermann JF, et al. Unmet needs of persons with cancer in Pennsylvania during the period of terminal care. *Cancer* 1988;62:627-34.
10. Canadian Cancer Society. *The final report on the needs of persons living with cancer across Canada.* Toronto: The Society; 1992.
11. Iscoe NA, Bruera E, Choo RC. Prostate cancer: 10. Palliative care. *CMAJ* 1999;160(3):365-71. [Chapter 10 in this book.]
12. Gray RE, Greenberg M, Fitch M, Parry N, Douglas MS, Labrecque M. Perspectives of cancer survivors interested in unconventional therapies. *J Psychosoc Oncol* 1997;15:149-71.
13. Hassouna MM, Heaton JPW. Prostate cancer: 8. Urinary incontinence and erectile dysfunction. *CMAJ* 1999;160(1):78-86. [Chapter 8 in this book.]
14. Gleave ME, Bruchovsky N, Moore MJ, Venner P. Prostate cancer: 9. Treatment of advanced disease. *CMAJ* 1999;160(2):225-32. [Chapter 9 in this book.]
15. Gray RE, Greenberg M, Fitch M, Sawka C, Hampson A, Labrecque M, et al. Information needs of women with metastatic breast cancer. *Cancer Prev Control* 1998;2(2):57-62.
16. Gray RE, Fitch M, Davis C, Phillips C. Interviews with men with prostate cancer about their self-help experience. *J Palliat Care* 1997;13:15-21.

Index

Page numbers in italic indicate that the information referred to is only in a figure or table on that page

A
acetaminophen 125
age
  as risk factor 2-7, *22*, 29
  and erectile capacity 92, 93
  and incidence rates 3
  and mortality rates 3
  of Canadian population 3, *4*, 5, 29, 143
  and prognosis 14-15
  and prostatectomy 58
  prostate-specific antigen (PSA) tests 47, 48
  table of probabilities 6-7
agricultural work 28
aircraft manufacturing industry 28
airline pilots 28
alpha-tocopherol *see* vitamin E
alprostadil *see* prostaglandin E1
alternative therapy *see* complementary therapy
American Cancer Society 36, 37
American College of Radiology 36
American Urological Association 29, 36, 79
analgesics
  to relieve pain 121, 125-26, 138
  to treat cystitis/urethritis 78
anatomy
  bladder outlet 84-85
  prostate region of pelvis *60*

androgen ablation
  combined therapies 106-7
  complications 108-9
  effectiveness 106, 138
  methods 103-4
  quality-of-life issues 108-9
  side effects 104, 105-6
  when to initiate 107-8
androgens 101-2
androstenedione 102
anorexia 126
anti-androgens 104-5, 106-7, 138
anti-angiogenesis therapy 140
antibiotics
  before prostatectomy 59-60
  to treat delirium 127
anticholinergics 87
antispasmodics 78, 79
anxiety 92
apomorphine *95*, 96
apoptosis stimulation 140
artificial urinary sphincter 88-89
Asia 21-22
autologous blood donation 59, 62
autologous fat 88

B
benign prostatic hyperplasia *22*, 27-28

beta-carotene 24, *34*
bicalutamide 105
biofeedback 87
biological treatments 140-41
biopsy
  about 36, 51-52
  recommendations 52-53
bisphosphonates 126, 140
bladder
  anatomy 84-85
  complications *75*, 76-77, 78-79
bladder-neck contracture
  after prostatectomy 64
  after radiation therapy *76*, 77
blood loss 62-63
body mass 26, 27
bone lesions 121-24
bone marrow failure 110
brachytherapy 73, 74-75, 136-37
breast cancer
  relation to prostate cancer 24
  screening sensitivity and specificity 37-38, 39
British Columbia, prostate cancer costs 147
bulking agents 88
buserelin 104

C

Canadian Cancer Society 6, 155
Canadian Prostate Cancer Network 6
cancer *see specific type or body part*
cardiac arrhythmia 62
catheterization
  after prostatectomy 61, 62
  after radiation therapy 74
  with radiation therapy 78
Caverject *see* prostaglandin E1
chemical workers 28
chemotherapy
  costs 148-49
  effectiveness 110-11, 120
  estramustine combinations 112
  mitoxantrone plus prednisone 111-12, 139
  suramin 112-13
  to relieve pain 139-40
China 21
clodronate 140
codeine
  causing delirium 127
  to relieve pain 125
collagen (bovine) with glutaraldehyde 88
colon cancer 24
combined androgen blockade 106-7
communication with patient 157-58, 160
comorbidity *14*, 15, 24
complementary therapy
  defined 118
  evaluating 118-21
complications
  costs 148
  prostatectomy 5, 58, 62-66
  radiation therapy 74, 75-79
computed tomography 51, 135-36
conformal radiotherapy 135-36
conservative management *see* "watchful waiting"
constipation 63, 127
continuity of care 159, 160-61
corticosteroids 126
cortisone 78, 79
costs
  defining 143-44
  direct 144-49
  effectiveness 149-51
  future trends 151
  indirect 144, 149
  prostate cancer compared with other diseases *145*
cryosurgery 132
CT *see* computed tomography
cyproterone acetate 105

D

deep venous thrombosis *62*, 63
dehydroepiandrosterone 102
delirium 125, 127-28
depression 92
Detrol *see* tolteridine
diabetes 92
diagnosis
  biopsy 51-52
  cost-effectiveness 151
  digital rectal examination 44
  importance of being early 43-44, 52-53
  prostate-specific antigen test 45-50
  transrectal ultrasonography 50-51
diarrhea
  after prostatectomy 63

after radiation therapy *75*, 79
diet
  after prostatectomy 61
  as risk factor *22*, 29
  complementary therapies 118
  fats 24, 25, *34*
  micronutrients 24, *34*
  selenium 25
  soy products 25-26
  tomato products 25
  vitamin E 24, 25
diethylstilbestrol 104-5, 108
digital rectal examination (DRE)
  about 44-45
  recommendations *45*, 52-53
  sensitivity and specificity 36, 37-38
dihydrotestosterone 102-3, 106
DRE *see* digital rectal examination (DRE)

E
edema
  after radiation therapy *76*, 78
  treatment 124-25
endometrial cancer 24
environment 5
erectile dysfunction
  after hormone therapy 92
  after prostatectomy 5, 64-65, 92-93
  after radiation therapy 5, *76*, 77, 79
  causes 91-92
  defined 90-91, 92
  prevention 78, 92-94
  quality of life 159
  treatment 94-97
erectile function
  and age 92, 93
  physiology 91
  and surgical methods 60-61
erythropoietin 59, 62-63
Essiac 118
estradiol 112
estramustine 112
etatsorp 119-21
ethnicity
  as risk factor 21-22, 27, 29
  and prognosis 11
etoposide 112

European Organization for Research and Treatment of Cancer 72, 112
European Randomized Study of Screening for Prostate Cancer 37, 39
expectant management *see* "watchful waiting"
external-beam radiation therapy 70-73, 75-78

F
family history 22-23, 29
farming work 28
fat (body) 26
fat (dietary)
  risk factor *22*, 24, 25
  studies *34*
fatigue
  after prostatectomy 63
  after radiation therapy 75, 79
  treatment 138-40
  with advanced cancer 110, 138
fentanyl
  causing delirium 127
  to relieve pain 125
Finland 25
flavoxate 87
fluoroscopy 86-87
flutamide
  for androgen ablation 105, 107
  withdrawal syndrome 106

G
gastrointestinal symptoms 16-17, 125
gene therapy 140
genetic risk factors *22*, 23-24, 29
genistein 25
geography 21-22
Gleason grading method *11*, 12-13
goserelin 104
gracilis myoplasty 89
grading of tumour *11*, 12-13
green tea 118

H
haloperidol 128
hematuria
  after prostatectomy 63
  after radiation therapy 79
  treatment 124

hemibody irradiation 120, 122-23
homeopathic therapy 119
Hoosier Oncology Group 112
hormonal factors 22, 26, 27, 29
hormone-refractory prostate cancer
  defined 110
  symptoms 110, 138-40
  treatment 110-14, 137-41
hormones 101-3
hormone therapy
  androgen ablation 103-9, 138
  complications 92, 108-9
  new approaches 138
  quality-of-life issues 108-9
  with palliative care 69
  with prostatectomy 59
  with radiation therapy 71-72, 78
hydration 127
hydrocortisone 113
hydromorphone
  causing delirium 127
  to relieve pain 125

I
imipramine 87
immune system therapies 118, 119-21, 140
impotence *see* erectile dysfunction
incidence, *see also* mortality
  age-specific 3
  age-standardized 3, 4
  Asia 21
  Canada 1-2, 21
  China 21
  compared to other cancers 1-2
  predicting 5-6
  province to province 3, 5
  Sweden 21
  United States 4, 6, 21
incontinence
  after prostatectomy 5, 63, 64-65, ˙, 85
  after radiation therapy 76, 77
  diagnosis 86-87
  quality of life 159-60
  treatment 87-89
  types 85-86
infection 62
inhibition of growth-factor receptors 140
interstitial brachytherapy 73, 74-75, 136-37

interstitial microwave thermoablation 132-35
iodine 125 74-75, 137
iridium 192 74-75

J
Japan
  dietary factors 25
  mortality rates 24

K
Kegel exercises 63-64, 65, 87-88

L
laxatives
  to relieve constipation 127
  to relieve nausea 127
leuprolide 104, 107
life expectancy, and treatment choice 16, 131
local-field radiotherapy 120, 121-22
luteinizing hormone-releasing hormone
  normal function 102
  suppressing 104-5
lycopenes 25
lymphadenopathy 125
lymphocele 62

M
magnetic resonance imaging 51
mammography 37-38, 39
megestrol
  for androgen ablation 105
  to stimulate appetite 126
meperidine 127
metabolism 11
metal product fabrication industry 28
methadone 127-28
metoclopramide 127
micronutrients 24, 34
midazolam 128
Milken, Michael 156
mind–body therapies 118
mitoxantrone
  to relieve pain 139
  to treat advanced cancer 111-12
morphine
  causing delirium 127
  to relieve pain 125

mortality, *see also* incidence
  age-specific 3
  associated with prostatectomy 58, 63
  costs 144, 149
  and ethnicity 24
  incidence 2-3, 5, 11
  lifetime risk 4
  predicting 5-6
  province to province 3, 5
  with conservative treatment 13
MRI *see* magnetic resonance imaging
MUSE *see* prostaglandin E1
myocardial infarction 62

N
National Cancer Institute
  combined androgen blockade 107
  pain studies 140
nausea 126-27
nerve root compression 124
Netherlands 145
nilutamide 105
normovolemic hemodilution 59, 62
nornitrogen mustard 112
Norway 145

O
obesity 26
occupational exposure 28
Ontario, prostate cancer costs 147, 148-49
opioid analgesics
  causing delirium 127
  to relieve pain 125-26
orchidectomy 103-4, 106-7, 138
oxybutynin 87
oxycodone
  causing delirium 127
  to relieve pain 125P

P
paclitaxel 112
pain
  after prostatectomy 61-62, 63
  from bone lesions 121-24, 138-39
  from spinal cord or nerve root compression 124
  treatment 124, 125-26, 138-40
  with advanced cancer 110
palladium 103 74-75, 137

palliative care
  complementary therapies 118-21
  radiotherapy 120, 121-25, 126, 138-39
  symptom control 125-28
papaverine 97
patient
  communication with 157-58, 160
  continuity of care 159, 160-61
  impatience 156, 157, 161
  participation in health care 155, 157, 161
  quality of life 13-14, 108-9, 158-60
  treatment choice 16-17, 69-70, 72, 79-80, 94, 111, 131
pelvic floor rehabilitation 63-64, 65, 87-88
penile prosthesis 94, *95*, 97
perfluorooctanoic acid 28
pharmacotherapy
  to treat erectile dysfunction 94-97
  to treat incontinence 87
phenazopyridine 78
phentolamine *95*, 96-97
phosphodiesterase inhibitors 96
physical activity
  after prostatectomy 63-64, 65
  as risk factor 26, 27
  and incontinence 86
  and prognosis 11
Physicians' Health Study (US) 40
physician's role
  continuity of care 160-61
  patient communication 157-58, 160-61
  PSA screening 156-57
  screening 36
polytetrafluoroethylene 88
prednisone
  to relieve pain 139
  to treat advanced cancer 111-12
preventive measures
  for cancer 22
  for erectile dysfunction 78, 92-94
proctitis *76*, 77, 78-79
progestational drugs 126
prognosis
  age factors 14-15
  assessing 10-14
  comorbidity *14*, 15
prolonged ileus 62
propantheline 87

prostaglandin E1 94-95, 96-97
prostate cancer
  burden
    economic 143-49, 151
    personal 4-5, 111
    societal 5, 7, 111, 149
  comorbidity *14*, 15, 24
  diagnostic tools 43-53, 151
  grading *11*, 12-13
  incidence 1-3, 4, 5-6, 21
  mortality rates 2-3, 5, 11
  natural history 9-14
  prevalence 2
  prognosis 10-15
  public awareness 6, 157
  risk factors 2-7, 21-29, *34*
  screening 35-41, 150, 156-57
  staging 13
  survival rates 72
  treatment
    biological approaches 139, 140-41
    chemotherapy 110-14
    complementary 118-21
    cryosurgery 132
    hormone therapy 103-9, 113-14, 138
    life expectancy 16
    palliative radiotherapy 120, 121-25, 126, 138-39
    prostatectomy 41, 57-67, 83, 84, 92-93
    radiation therapy 69-80, 135-37
    symptom control 125-28, 138-40
    thermoablation 132-35
    watchful waiting 10-14, 16-17, 57-58, 69
prostatectomy
  candidates 58
  complications 58, 59, 62-66, 92-93
  defined 57
  figures *60*, *61*
  follow-up 41, 66-67
  increasing rate 83
  mortality 58, 63
  nerve-sparing 60-61, 92-93
  patient preparation 59-60
  post-surgical hospitalization 61-62
  procedures 58-59, 60-61, 84
  radical 59, 132

prostate-specific antigen (PSA) test
  about 44, 45-46
  after prostatectomy 66
  age-specific ranges 47, 48
  evaluating 36, 40-41
  introduced 2, 5, 36
  limitations 50
  patient education 156-57
  percentage of free PSA 49-50
  PSA density 46-47
  PSA velocity 48-49
  recommendations 44, 52-53
  sensitivity and specificity 36, 37-38
  United States 4, 6
prostatic acid phosphatase test 45
prosthesis, penile 94, *95*, 97
public awareness 6, 157
pulmonary embolism *62*, 63
pyridium 78

Q

quality of life
  and androgen ablation 108-9
  patient's view 158-60
  and prognosis 13-14
Quebec, prostate cancer costs 147

R

radiation therapy
  complication management 78-79
  complications 74, 75-78
  conformal 135-36
  contraindications 80
  dose 72-73
  external-beam 70-73, 75-78, 120, 121
  failure 135
  indications 79-80
  interstitial brachytherapy 73, 74-75, 136-37
  outlook 137
  palliative 120, 121-25, 126
  survival rates 70-71
Radiation Therapy Oncology Group 72, 73, 77
radical perineal prostatectomy 59
radical retropubic prostatectomy 59
radionecrosis 78
railway transport workers 28

rectal complications
  prostatectomy 59, *62*, 63
  radiation therapy *75*, *76*, 77, 78-79
risk factors
  age 2, 3-7, *22*, 29
  benign prostatic hyperplasia *22*, 27-28
  body mass 26, 27
  diet *22*, 24-26, 29, *34*
  environmental 5
  ethnicity 11, 21-22, 27, 29
  family history 22-23, 29
  genetic *22*, 23-24, 29
  geographic 21-22
  hormonal *22*, 26-27, 29
  lifetime 3-7
  metabolism 11
  occupation 28
  physical activity 11, 26, 27
  preventive measures *22*
  sexual history *22*, 27
  smoking 11
  table of probabilities 6-7
  vasectomy *22*, 26, 27

S

Saskatchewan, prostate cancer costs 147
screening
  cost-effectiveness 150
  defined 35-36, 157
  evaluation of programs 38
  evaluation of tests 36-38
  ongoing trials 39-41
  value 39, 156-57
  World Health Organization criteria 40
selenium 25
self-help groups 160-61
sexual dysfunction 80
sexual history *22*, 27
sildenafil 95-96
silicone 88
sitz baths 78
skeletal metastatic lesions 121-24
smoking
  erectile dysfunction 92
  and prognosis 11
soy products 25-26
spinal cord compression 124
staging of tumour 13

stress 92
strontium 89 120, 123-24, 139
structural metal erector industry 28
support groups 160-61
suramin 112-13
surgery
  cryosurgery 132
  implant to treat incontinence 88-89
  interstitial microwave thermoablation 132-35
  orchidectomy 103-4, 106-7, 138
  prostatectomy 41, 57-67, 83, 84, 92-93
  spinal cord decompression 124
  thermoablation 132
Sweden
  incidence 21
  prostate cancer costs 145
systemic radionuclide therapy 120, 123-24

T

TAP *see* apomorphine
Teflon *see* polytetrafluoroethylene
testosterone 102-3
thermoablation 132-35
thrombosis *62*, 63
tolteridine 87
tomato products 25
transrectal ultrasonography (TRUS)
  about 36, 50-51
  recommendations *45*, 53
  screening studies 37-38
  to guide brachytherapy 137
trazodone *95*
treatment
  androgen ablation 103-6
  brachytherapy 136-37
  choice of 16-17, 69-70, 94, 111
  complementary therapies 118-21
  conformal radiotherapy 135-36
  cost 144-49
  cost effectiveness 150-51
  cryosurgery 132
  evaluating 118-21, 156
  hormone therapy 59, 69
  palliative radiotherapy 120, 121-25, 126, 138-39
  patient choice 16-17, 69-70, 72, 79-80, 94, 111, 131
  radiation therapy 69-80

surgery 57-67
symptom control 125-28
thermoablation 132-35
watchful waiting 10-14, 16-17, 57-58, 69
TRUS *see* transrectal ultrasonography (TRUS)

U

ultrasonography *see* transrectal ultrasonography
unconventional therapy *see* complementary therapy
United States
  complementary therapies 118
  incidence 4, 6, 21
  new radiotherapies 135
  prostate cancer costs 145-46
  screening 4, 6, 36
ureteral injury 62
ureteric obstruction 124
urethral stricture 76, 77
urinary incontinence *see* incontinence
urodynamic study 86-87

US National Cancer Institute 36

V

vacuum erection devices 94, *95*
vasectomy 22, 26, 27
vasoactive intestinal polypeptide with phentolamine 96
Vasomax *see* phentolamine
Viagra *see* sildenafil
vinblastine 112
vitamin A 24, *34*
vitamin E 24, 25

W

"watchful waiting"
  contraindicated 57-58
  defined 10
  patient choice 16-17, 69
  studies 10-14
water-transport industry 28
weight loss 110
World Health Organization screening criteria 40
worry 92

Y

yohimbine *95*